Prehospital Research Methods and Practice

Edited by

Aloysius Niroshan Siriwardena and Gregory Adam Whitley

Disclaimer

Class Professional Publishing have made every effort to ensure that the information, tables, drawings and diagrams contained in this book are accurate at the time of publication. The book cannot always contain all the information necessary for determining appropriate care and cannot address all individual situations; therefore, individuals using the book must ensure they have the appropriate knowledge and skills to enable suitable interpretation. Class Professional Publishing does not guarantee, and accepts no legal liability of whatever nature arising from or connected to, the accuracy, reliability, currency or completeness of the content of *Prehospital Research Methods and Practice*. Users must always be aware that such innovations or alterations after the date of publication may not be incorporated in the content. Please note, however, that Class Professional Publishing assumes no responsibility whatsoever for the content of external resources in the text or accompanying online materials.

The information presented in this book is accurate and current to the best of the authors' knowledge.

The authors and publisher, however, make no guarantee as to, and assume no responsibility for, the correctness, sufficiency or completeness of such information or recommendation.

Printing history

This edition first published in 2022

The authors and publisher welcome feedback from the users of this book. Please contact the publisher:

Class Professional Publishing,

The Exchange, Express Park, Bristol Road, Bridgwater TA6 4RR

Telephone: 01278 472 800

Email: post@class.co.uk

Website: www.classprofessional.co.uk

Class Professional Publishing is an imprint of Class Publishing Ltd

A CIP catalogue record for this book is available from the British Library

Paperback ISBN: 9781859599808

eBook ISBN: 9781859599792

Cover design by Hybert Design Limited, UK

Designed and typeset by S4Carlisle Publishing Services

Printed in the UK by Cambrian Printers Ltd

This book is printed on paper from responsible sources. Refer to local recycling guidance on disposal of this book.

Contents

Contents

Contents

Chapter 5: Experimental and Quasi-experimental Designs   111

Gavin Perkins, Chen Ji and Mike Smyth

Chapter 10: Quality Improvement 207

David M. Williams

List of Figures

List of Tables

List of Boxes

About the Authors

Stephanie Armstrong PhD

Stephanie Armstrong is a Senior Lecturer at the University of Lincoln. She has a diverse academic background, having originally completed her PhD in Behavioural Ecology focusing on zoo animals. A change of direction led to the subsequent completion of degrees in forensic anthropology and medical herbalism. She initially joined the University of Lincoln as the researcher on the Network exploring Ethics of Ambulance Trials (NEAT) project and has extensive experience as a Research Ethics Board reviewer. Her current research is grounded in healthcare improvement, focusing particularly on mental health provision in Lower- and Middle-Income Countries.

Ffion Curtis PhD

Ffion Curtis is the Academic Lead for the Centre for Ethnic Health Research within the National Institute for Health Research (NIHR) Applied Research Collaboration (ARC) East Midlands. Ffion has experience of working collaboratively across a broad range of populations, contexts and methodologies, with her research predominantly focusing on ethnicity and health inequalities, and the role of lifestyle and behavioural interventions in the prevention and management of chronic conditions. After completing her PhD titled 'The Role of Vitamin D and Physical Activity in Glycaemic Homeostasis' at Aberystwyth University in 2013, she continued her work in diabetes, conducting a feasibility study of a peer-led diabetes self-management programme within Hywel Dda University Health Board (Wales). Ffion then spent several years at the University of Lincoln, where she developed and led the Lincoln Institute for Health Systematic Review Training Programme for academics and NHS colleagues working across the East Midlands. She has experience of conducting systematic reviews (quantitative, qualitative and mixed methods) in a wide range of areas relating to public health and clinical research, many of which are being used to underpin both research and practice.

Chen Ji PhD

Chen Ji is an Associate Professor in Clinical Trial Statistics at Warwick Clinical Trials Unit, Warwick Medical School, the University of Warwick. He mainly works in emergency and critical care trials and rehabilitation trials funded by the National Institute for Health Research. His research interests include the development and application of new methodologies related to clinical research.

Adèle Langlois PhD
Adèle Langlois is Associate Professor at the University of Lincoln. She has degrees in biological anthropology and international relations. Her PhD explored the global governance of bioethics and human genetics, particularly at UNESCO. She held a Wellcome Trust Biomedical Ethics Fellowship at the Parliamentary Office of Science and Technology as part of her doctoral studies, during which she wrote a policy briefing on research ethics in developing countries. Adèle joined the University of Lincoln in September 2009. She is the author of *Negotiating Bioethics: The Governance of the UNESCO Bioethics Programme* (Routledge, 2013). She has also worked on ethics governance in prehospital research as Co-Investigator on the Wellcome-funded Network exploring Ethics of Ambulance Trials (NEAT) project, and is currently researching regulatory bottlenecks in global health.

Despina Laparidou MSc
Despina Laparidou has been a health services researcher at the Community and Health Research Unit (CaHRU) within the University of Lincoln since 2014. Her background is in psychology and she has training in research methods in psychology (UK), health psychology (UK) and cognitive behavioural therapy (Greece). Despina has conducted research in a variety of areas, including dementia, diabetes and ambulance services. She has conducted quantitative, qualitative systematic and mixed methods reviews in areas such as insomnia, autism, tinnitus, robotic and robot-assisted interventions in motor rehabilitation, as well as educational interventions for informal carers of people with dementia.

Bill Lord PhD
Bill Lord is a registered paramedic, educator and researcher who worked as a paramedic in Sydney, Melbourne and more recently with the Queensland Ambulance Service until 2018. He has worked in higher education for 25 years, including at Charles Sturt University where he was a Senior Lecturer and coordinator of the Bachelor of Clinical Practice (Paramedic) programme. In 2004, he was appointed to the position of Head of Undergraduate Paramedic Programs at Monash University and in 2012 moved to the University of the Sunshine Coast to take up the position of Associate Professor and Discipline Leader for Paramedic Science until 2019. Research interests include the development of critical thinking and diagnostic reasoning skills in novice paramedics, work-integrated learning and pain management in the out-of-hospital setting. Bill currently has an adjunct Associate Professor appointment within the Department of Paramedicine at Monash University.

Alicia O'Cathain PhD
Alicia O'Cathain is Professor of Health Services Research at the School of Health and Related Research at the University of Sheffield. She is also a Senior Investigator at the National Institute of Health Research. She leads research on emergency and urgent care, evaluation of new health services, and the development and evaluation of complex interventions for chronic conditions and methodology. Her emergency and urgent care research has focused on understanding demand for emergency ambulances and emergency departments, outcomes important to emergency

ambulance service users, evaluation of new services (such as NHS 111) and explaining variation in practice (for example, emergency admissions and ambulance non-conveyance). She has written extensively about how to do mixed methods research, focusing on quality, integration and reporting of this important approach. In 2018, she published the book *A Practical Guide to Using Qualitative Research with Randomized Controlled Trials* (Oxford University Press). Recently, she has published MRC-funded guidance on intervention development and runs short courses on this topic.

Dayne O'Meara PhD

Dayne O'Meara is an anthropologist who received his PhD from The Australian National University in 2020. From the start of 2017 to mid-2018, he conducted long-term ethnographic research with the Sgaw Karen people in the north of Thailand. He has worked closely with children of all ages to research topics related to education, poverty, gender, development, ethnic discrimination and national identity politics. His PhD thesis, *Disciplining the Heart: Love, School, and Growing Up Karen in Mae Hong Son*, presents the extended case study of a lower secondary school student who was expelled and then married following a romantic affair. He has experience implementing a wide range of qualitative methods beyond formal interviews, including film, photography, play, drawing and participant observation. He is currently working as an anthropologist for the Northern Land Council in Darwin, Australia, where he conducts archival and ethnographic genealogical research to help secure the rights and interests of Indigenous Australians in relation to the Aboriginal Land Rights Act and the Native Title Act of Australia.

Peter O'Meara PhD

Peter O'Meara is an Adjunct Professor in the Monash University Department of Paramedicine in Australia. Peter is an internationally recognised expert on paramedicine models and was one of the first paramedics in the world to complete a doctorate, in which he used mixed methods and soft systems methodology to research rural paramedic systems. He is a nationally registered paramedic and a Fellow of the Australasian College of Paramedicine, with academic qualifications in health administration, public policy and agricultural health and medicine. Dr O'Meara has used a wide range of research methodologies, from randomised control trials to ethnography, to explore clinical questions, undertake health services research and explore the development of innovative paramedic roles. Peter's research interest has shifted towards the professionalisation of paramedicine, and violence against health workers. He has published one book, 12 book chapters, 88 peer-reviewed papers and other articles in professional publications. His body of work continues to influence the growth of paramedicine as a health profession. Dr O'Meara is a member of several graduate research student supervisory teams across four universities, with his students located in three countries. Peter is an Associate Editor of the *Australasian Journal of Paramedicine* and a member of the Journal Advisory Committee of the *Australian Journal of Rural Health*. He has been an Expert Assessor for the Australian Research Council and has peer reviewed for the Emergency Medicine Foundation in Australia and the New Frontiers in Research Fund in Canada.

Gavin Perkins MD

Gavin Perkins is Professor of Critical Care Medicine and Director of Warwick Clinical Trials Unit, based at Warwick Medical School within the University of Warwick. He holds honorary appointments as a Consultant Physician with University Hospitals Birmingham (critical care) and West Midlands Ambulance Service (MERIT Consultant). He is a Fellow of the Academy of Medical Sciences and a National Institute for Health Research Senior Investigator. He has been the chief investigator for several National Institute for Health Research-funded prehospital trials, including the PARAMEDIC, PARAMEDIC2, PARAMEDIC3 and RePHILL trials. He is co-chair of the International Liaison Committee on Resuscitation, Director of Science for the European Resuscitation Council (incorporating the ERC Research NET) and chairs the Resuscitation Council UK Community and Ambulance Committee.

Tom Quinn MPhil

Tom Quinn is a nurse with four decades of experience in cardiovascular care. His career includes working in hospital and prehospital settings, the latter as a consultant cardiac nurse, and in a government policy team responsible for cardiovascular strategy. He is professor of cardiovascular nursing at Kingston University & St George's, University of London, undertaking collaborative research in cardiac arrest and acute cardiovascular care. He has published extensively, including studies funded by the British Heart Foundation and the National Institute for Health Research, and has supervised several paramedics undertaking PhD studies. He is a member of the UK's Joint Royal Colleges Ambulance Liaison Committee, leading on acute coronary syndrome and stroke guidelines. He is a Fellow of the Royal College of Nursing, European Society of Cardiology, American Heart Association and American College of Cardiology. In 2019, he was elected Honorary Fellow of the College of Paramedics. Tom is a non-executive director of a large NHS ambulance service, Trustee of the British Association for Immediate Care and his volunteer roles include serving as a board member for the European Society of Cardiology Association for Acute Cardiovascular Care and locally promoting CPR and public access defibrillation.

Aloysius Niroshan Siriwardena PhD

Niroshan (Niro) Siriwardena is Professor of Primary and Prehospital Health Care at the University of Lincoln. He is director of the Community and Health Research Unit at the University of Lincoln, a research centre which focuses on quality improvement and implementation research, including studies aimed at development and evaluation of quality measures and health technologies in primary care and ambulance services. He is also director of the Lincoln Clinical Trials Unit, an Honorary Professor at Cardiff University and board member of the 999 EMS Research Forum. He trained in medicine at St. Bartholomew's Hospital Medical College London and in general practice in Lincolnshire, followed by research training at Nottingham and De Montfort Universities. He has published over 130 research studies, including the Prehospital Outcomes for Evidence Based Evaluation research programme, in leading journals, including funding from the National Institute for Health Research, Research Councils UK, the Health Foundation and the Wellcome Trust.

Mike Smyth PhD

Mike Smyth is a critical care paramedic and Assistant Professor in Emergency and Critical Care at Warwick Clinical Trials Unit, part of Warwick Medical School, at the University of Warwick. Mike is co-chief investigator for the National Institute for Health Research-funded PACKMaN and PROTECTeD studies. He is vice-chair of the Basic Life Support Task Force of the International Liaison Committee on Resuscitation, a member of the Basic Life Support Science and Education Committee of the European Resuscitation Council and a board member of the 999 EMS Research Committee.

Gregory Adam Whitley PhD

Gregory Adam Whitley is a paramedic research fellow with the East Midlands Ambulance Service NHS Trust (EMAS) and a lecturer in paramedic science at the University of Lincoln. He joined the ambulance service in 2010 and has been a registered paramedic since 2012. During 2015–2017, he worked on the National Institute for Health Research (NIHR)-funded AIRWAYS-2 clinical trial as a research paramedic for EMAS. In 2020, he completed his PhD, funded by the NIHR Applied Research Collaboration – East Midlands (ARC-EM), on the topic of prehospital pain management in children. He joined the *British Paramedic Journal* in May 2021 as an associate editor and is currently undertaking a post-doctoral bridging fellowship funded by Health Education England.

David M. Williams PhD

David M. Williams is an independent consultant at DavidMWilliamsPhD.com. He is a scholar-practitioner of the science of improvement and a subject matter expert on ambulance system design and improvement. He also serves as a senior improvement advisor and subject matter expert on ambulance systems and care to the Institute for Healthcare Improvement (IHI). Previously a member of the IHI leadership team, he led IHI's global Improvement Science and Methods and Leadership work. He started his career as a volunteer firefighter and worked as a paramedic in cities across the United States. Previously, leadership roles included Commander for the Austin/Travis County EMS in Austin, Texas, and an international ambulance system consultant for an international firm. He has published several book chapters and dozens of articles on ambulance topics. He co-developed and published two peer-reviewed papers on the EMS Trigger Tool to Measure Adverse Events. He earned a BS in EMS Management and an MS in Emergency Health Services Management. He also earned a PhD in Organizational Systems, where his research focused on the obstacles to patient-centric EMS system design. Dr Williams serves on the Advisory Board of the Austin/Travis County EMS in Austin, Texas.

Foreword

It is a privilege to write a short Foreword to this book on *Prehospital Research Methods and Practice*. The topic is a crucial one, not least because the majority of *unexpected* deaths occur at home, and comparatively few in hospital.

But other issues are also fundamental and well addressed in the book. Ethical issues are very important. Gaining consent is not always possible, and if obtained it is often beset by misunderstandings. It is good to see respect for autonomy, non-maleficence, beneficence and justice emphasised, together with the need for systematic reviews, preferably conducted by multidisciplinary groups.

Another accentuated aim is to avoid misleading readers with incomplete or inaccurate quotations. Stressed too is the avoidance of language that could cause confusion by variations in its usage between countries.

The book makes a valuable contribution to a very important topic.

Professor Douglas Chamberlain

Preface

We are pleased to introduce this new text on *Prehospital Research Methods and Practice*. It has been a privilege to conceive this volume and to bring together a distinguished group of leading international experts in the fields of prehospital, ambulance, Emergency Medical Services (EMS) and urgent care research, from the UK, Australia and the USA, as contributors and authors. We are honoured that Professor Douglas Chamberlain, the father of modern paramedicine who celebrated his 90th birthday last year (2021) and who first trained paramedics in resuscitation in Brighton, England in the 1970s, has kindly provided the Foreword.

The main rationale for this book was to provide an accessible and up-to-date textbook, broadly covering applied research methods in this important and rapidly advancing research setting, to meet the needs of undergraduate and postgraduate students in paramedic science, medicine, nursing or allied health, who are interested in undertaking research in the prehospital and ambulance setting. It is designed to meet the needs of the paramedicine, emergency medicine and wider healthcare communities, explaining and illustrating key approaches, through recent examples of work undertaken by the authors and other researchers working in this field.

When we began working in the prehospital research field over 20 years ago, ambulance research was still in its infancy. Ambulance services and clinicians needed and wanted an evidence base that was developed in the EMS setting and which supported their work and academic standing among the clinical professions.

To achieve this, there was a need to develop the infrastructure for multicentre research involving ambulance services, to overcome the logistical problems of study delivery, for example related to acquiring and linking data for observational studies and to solve problems of recruitment, randomisation and consent for experimental approaches. Decisions on the priorities for prehospital research were needed and these were first published around a decade ago.

There was also a need to develop and support a cadre of excellent undergraduate and postgraduate research students working in prehospital research. This has come to fruition as evidenced by the growing numbers of doctoral students and completions recorded on the Paramedic PhD website (https://www.paramedicphd .com/), which was set up by Dr Greg Whitley whilst undertaking his doctorate.

Prehospital research has benefitted from its multi- and inter-disciplinary nature. Our contributing authors, who include clinical academic paramedics, emergency physicians, general practitioners and health services researchers, have been at the forefront of ambulance service research and, with others, have helped advance this field of research in leaps and bounds over the past two decades. Over this time, researchers have developed a range of patient-centred clinical outcome measures and indicators, have evaluated existing or novel interventions and pathways and have advanced multicentre trials for ambulance services. Through research supervision and training, many of our authors have also encouraged, trained and supported new researchers in this area of study, laying foundations for the future.

This endeavour would not have been possible without the support of others. In particular, we would like to thank our contributing authors who have done an extraordinary job of providing clear, accessible and expertly written chapters. Lianne Sherlock, senior editor at Class who originally encouraged the text, has provided helpful guidance and support throughout. We are also grateful to our colleagues in the Community and Health Research Unit at the University of Lincoln for providing feedback on chapters, particularly Professor Graham Law, Dr Vanessa Botan and Dr Elise Rowan. Finally, our families, friends and colleagues have provided encouragement and help throughout.

Aloysius Niroshan Siriwardena and Gregory Adam Whitley

Chapter 1

Introduction

Gregory Adam Whitley and Aloysius Niroshan Siriwardena

Chapter Objectives

This chapter will cover:

- The definition of research and an explanation of its importance for prehospital and paramedic practice
- Theory and evidence-based practice
- Advances in prehospital research
- Clinical audit and quality improvement
- Explanation of the research process from initial idea to dissemination
- Areas for future development

What is Research?

Research is the:

> 'creative and systematic work undertaken in order to increase the stock of knowledge'
>
> (OECD, 2015).

Research is *creative*: it is as much an art as it is a science. Answering a research question requires the development of a comprehensive research project, which involves selecting the appropriate research team, study design, population, data collection techniques and methods of analysis; this all requires creativity. The development of novel methods and innovative use of existing methods also require creativity.

Research is *systematic*: following the prescribed steps of published methods and careful consideration of published guidelines are important to maintain rigour. **Systematic reviews** (discussed in **Chapter 3: Systematic Reviews**) and **randomised controlled trials** (discussed in **Chapter 5: Experimental and Quasi-experimental Designs**) have robust guidelines and reporting standards, which should be followed to maintain quality (Moher et al., 2009; Schulz et al., 2010).

Research should *increase the stock of knowledge*: this should allow gaps in the evidence base to be addressed, answer important research questions or create a deeper understanding of complex clinical problems. A problem for researchers is that with more than 1,000,000 articles added to the PubMed database every year (Landhuis, 2016), it is becoming increasingly challenging to manage and synthesise the ever-growing volume of research. When searching PubMed (on 18 April 2021) for 'prehospital' in the year 2000 and 2020, the number of articles found were 235 and 1,887, respectively (an 800% increase in 20 years). Whilst increasing the stock of knowledge is desirable and to be encouraged, we need careful consideration of how the increasing volume of research will be managed effectively, so that important research is implemented into clinical practice to improve patient **outcomes**.

If research increases the stock of knowledge, it is important to briefly consider: what is knowledge? This question relates to the division of philosophy called **epistemology**, which simply refers to the nature of knowledge, and asks questions such as 'how can we know anything with any certainty?', 'must we have evidence to know the truth?', 'what are the limits of knowledge?' and 'how is knowledge acquired?'. The nature of knowledge has been debated for thousands of years, going back to the birth of Western philosophy in ancient Greece during the time of Socrates (470–399 BCE), Plato (429–347 BCE) and Aristotle (384–322 BCE). When we start to question our own knowledge, uncertainty arises. Some may find this concerning. Remember, it is better to be uncertain than overconfident. As Richard Feynman once said:

'I can live with doubt, and uncertainty, and not knowing. I think it's much more interesting, to live not knowing than to have answers which might be wrong'

(The Pleasure of Finding Things Out, 1981).

Why is Research Important?

How can we know anything with any certainty? This is an important question to consider when determining the importance of research. Clinicians develop experience during their practice. The longer they practise, the more experience they gain. Over time, clinicians develop opinions about which interventions are effective or not. This is referred to as anecdote and is highly dependent on the exposure of the clinician to various patients and conditions. Anecdotal evidence is useful, especially when there is a paucity of research evidence. However, it is highly biased because the clinician may have been exposed to an unrepresentative group of patients. This may lead them to develop opinions about that group of patients that do not accurately reflect the group at the population level. This means that their opinion may not be useful to inform national guidelines for example.

The **hierarchy of evidence** is useful to consider here. Many variations of the evidence hierarchy exist; see **Figure 1.1** for a standard example.

There are several problems with standard hierarchy of evidence illustrations, as shown in the example provided in **Figure 1.1**. They often do not show the full range of study

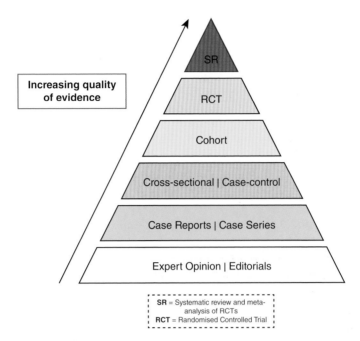

Figure 1.1 – Hierarchy of evidence.

types, such as qualitative or mixed methods studies, nor other types of reviews such as systemic reviews of qualitative studies, literature reviews or **rapid reviews**. These figures do have a simple purpose; they illustrate that in general, as the level of evidence increases from expert opinion to more advanced, robust research methods, the quality of evidence (**validity** and **reliability**) also increases. Validity generally relates to how closely the findings of a study represent the 'truth', and includes the notion of **internal validity**, that is, does the study show what it purports to, and **external validity**, that is, are the findings generalisable, for example: would the findings of a survey of 25 adults suffering diabetes represent the entire adult diabetic population of the UK? This would be extremely unlikely. Reliability generally relates to the repeatability of a study; if it were to be repeated, would the same findings be generated?

A single clinician's expert opinion is unlikely to have high validity or reliability; however, a clinical trial of airway management strategies for out-of-hospital cardiac arrest **enrolling** 9,296 patients across England (Benger et al., 2018) would have much higher validity and reliability. This simple example explains why research is important.

We need high-quality, robust evidence to inform prehospital clinical practice to ensure patients receive optimum care. We need to constantly challenge *current* clinical practice and ask difficult questions, such as 'does this adrenaline I'm giving to my patient with cardiac arrest cause more harm than good?'. The PARAMEDIC2 trial aimed to answer this clinical question, and concluded that the use of adrenaline in out-of-hospital cardiac arrest increased rates of 30-day survival, but did not increase rates of survival with favourable neurological outcome because more survivors had severe neurologic impairment in the adrenaline group (Perkins et al., 2018). This finding has challenged decades of paramedic practice in which adrenaline has been routinely used as part of paramedic practice.

We need to ask questions about *new* medical devices, such as 'which is the most effective airway management strategy for out-of-hospital cardiac arrest, a strategy of i-gel or tracheal tube first?'. The AIRWAYS-2 trial aimed to answer this and found no significant difference between strategies (Benger et al., 2018). The results of AIRWAYS-2 have influenced the debate about which airway device is better and have reduced the need for paramedics to routinely use tracheal tubes with their risks of injury or incorrect placement.

We also need to ask questions about other new *health technologies*, such as 'do mechanical chest compression devices improve survival in out-of-hospital cardiac arrest compared to manual chest compressions?'. The PARAMEDIC trial aimed to answer this and found no significant difference between the LUCAS-2 device and manual chest compressions (Perkins et al., 2015). Although external cardiac compression devices are still being used in out-of-hospital cardiac arrest, their use is largely limited to specific situations, such as prolonged resuscitation efforts or during ambulance transport.

Research is also important for the professionalisation of ambulance services and the paramedic profession. Civilian ambulance services were first created in the 1860s in the UK and US (Caroline, 2007; Ciottone, 2006), the 1880s in Canada (Ontario Paramedic Association, 2015) and the 1890s in Australia (Ambulance Service of New South Wales, 2018; Queensland Ambulance Service, 2018). The birth of the modern paramedic occurred in the late 1960s and early 1970s (Caroline, 2007; Chamberlain, 2018; White et al., 1973). Ambulance services have developed significantly since the late 19th century and have moved away from the traditional transport model where ambulance personnel were viewed as 'drivers' (Newton, 2012). In England during 2017, in 38% of calls to ambulance services attended by an ambulance, the patient was not transported to hospital (Coster et al., 2019). This illustrates the paradigm shift in prehospital clinical care that has occurred over the last 50 years.

As ambulance services and clinicians become more advanced and focused on patient satisfaction and outcomes, the more urgent is the need for high-quality, prehospital research to inform clinical practice. Prehospital research is important for the professionalisation of ambulance services and clinicians, and high-quality research specific to the prehospital setting is needed to improve patient outcomes.

Theory and Evidence-based Practice

Theory

All research is framed by theory, whether it is made explicit or not (Green and Thorogood, 2018). The use of theory within research should strengthen the purpose or rationale for conducting the research (Green, 2014; Lederman and Lederman, 2015) and is useful in helping to place research within broader fields of knowledge, aiding validity and contributing to **generalisability**/transferability (Green and Thorogood, 2018).

Different levels of theory exist, including macro/grand theory and middle-range theory. Macro/grand theories are formulated at a high level of abstraction and make broad generalisations that apply across many domains at a global level (Davidoff et al., 2015). Middle-range theories act as an intermediate, and link grand theory to minor working hypotheses (Davidoff et al., 2015).

We discussed earlier the concept of epistemology (the branch of philosophy concerned with the nature of knowledge). There is also a branch of philosophy concerned with the nature of reality; this is called **ontology**. When a researcher adopts a set of beliefs about the nature of reality (ontology) and the nature of knowledge (epistemology), they are said to have adopted a *paradigm*. This constitutes macro/grand theory, as it relates to the very nature of reality and knowledge through which we conduct research. Broadly speaking, there are two extremes of the spectrum when considering paradigms: **positivism/postpositivism** and **interpretivist/constructivist** (Guba and Lincoln, 1994). The literature on **research paradigms** is overwhelmingly extensive; many paradigms are not discussed here, and the aim is simply to provide a rudimentary introduction to the concept of research paradigms.

Positivism and Postpositivism

The nature of reality within the positivist paradigm argues that there is one reality and it is apprehendable. It is entirely separate from the observer and can be observed objectively. This leads into the nature of knowledge within the positivist paradigm: objectivist. Under the positivist paradigm, it is believed that reality can be observed in a purely objective manner, free from culture, personal beliefs and assumptions. A useful visualisation of positivism, according to Alderson (1998), is a scientist looking through a microscope; this represents the distance between the observer and observed and the resultant exclusion of the surrounding context, along with the use of reliable, visible 'hard' data.

In recent years, the positivist paradigm has been largely replaced by postpositivism, a paradigm founded by Bhaskar (1975), which is often used in healthcare research as it relies less on realism and objectivity and more on critical realism and modified objectivism (Guba and Lincoln, 1994). Postpositivism accepts that knowledge is conjectural, that is, subject to conjecture (an opinion or conclusion formed on the basis of incomplete information) (Phillips et al., 2000; Popper, 1962). The belief is that replicated findings are probably true, but are always subject to falsification (Guba and Lincoln, 1994). According to Karl Popper:

> 'There are no ultimate sources of knowledge. Every source, every suggestion, is welcome; and every source, every suggestion, is open to critical examination'
>
> (Popper, 1962).

This statement resonates well within the postpositivist paradigm as it accepts the use of multiple types of research, including quantitative and qualitative.

It might be clear at this point that the positivist and postpositivist paradigms are very much suited to quantitative methods, as discussed in **Chapter 4: Observational Studies** and **Chapter 5: Experimental and Quasi-experimental Designs**, whilst postpositivism is also suited to **mixed methods research** (Creswell, 2014), which is discussed in **Chapter 7: Mixed Methods Research**.

Interpretivism/Constructivism

Within the interpretivist/constructivist paradigm, it is argued that there are multiple realities, instead of one single reality as believed under positivism. This is because each individual person generates their own version of the world, from the day they are born, throughout their entire life. All their experiences, perceptions and beliefs have led them to create a version of reality that is their own, and no one else can share or experience their reality.

The ontology of the interpretivist/constructivist paradigm is something called relativism; reality is relative to each individual, and therefore the belief that multiple realities exist holds. The beliefs around the nature of knowledge within this paradigm are subjective (subjectivism) and knowledge is considered co-constructed between participant and researcher – and this intersubjectivity is fostered and valued (Weaver and Olson, 2006).

At this end of the 'paradigm spectrum', it might be clear that researchers adopting an interpretivist/constructivist paradigm are suited to qualitative research methods, where an understanding of participants' experiences, values and beliefs is needed to understand healthcare problems. Qualitative methods are discussed further in **Chapter 6: Qualitative Research**.

Having discussed the two major paradigms within healthcare research, and their subsequent lean towards quantitative or qualitative methods, you might ask what paradigms are used for mixed methods research. It is beyond the scope of this text to explore this further, but Tashakkori and Teddlie (2010) put forward interesting arguments regarding the contemporary issue of paradigms in mixed methods research and we advise this for further reading.

Evidence-based Practice

Evidence-based practice has been defined as:

> 'the conscientious, explicit, and judicious use of current best evidence in making decisions about the care of individual patients. The practice of evidence-based medicine means integrating individual clinical expertise with the best available external clinical evidence from systematic research'

> (Sackett et al., 1996).

This definition considers the best available evidence (produced by researchers) and clinical expertise (acquired by clinicians) but doesn't fully embrace patient values and preferences. Whilst an intervention may be evidence based, and there may be a need for it based on clinical experience, it might not be preferable or acceptable for some patients. Interventions should be developed using patient and public involvement and engagement (PPIE). There is increasing recognition of the benefits of PPIE, and methods of co-creation and co-production are of increasing interest (Voorberg et al., 2015).

There are three important aspects of evidence-based practice: best available evidence, clinical experience and patient values and preferences; see **Figure 1.2** for the model of evidence-based practice.

Evidence-based practice has been beneficial to patients and practitioners over the last 20 years by informing and ensuring high-quality clinical practice and reducing or stopping the wasteful use of ineffective or potentially harmful treatments. The volume of evidence in the prehospital setting has increased significantly, resulting in the removal of once-common practices. Such practices included routine administration of supplemental oxygen for heart attack patients, applying rigid cervical collars to most road traffic collision patients and regularly administering paracetamol to reduce pyrexia. These once-common practices have been deemed to lack benefit and in some cases to be harmful (Sundstrøm et al., 2014). It is extremely important that as the body of evidence grows due to the increasing number of prehospital studies, services and clinicians keep up to date to continue providing optimum care to patients.

Remember that all evidence is not created equally, and due diligence is required when evaluating evidence for its quality. This is covered in **Chapter 9: Critically Appraising a Paper and Preparing a Paper for Publication** and is essential reading

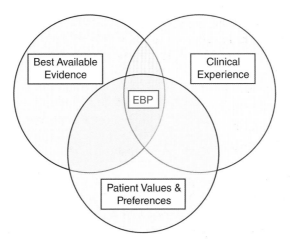

Figure 1.2 – Evidence-based practice model.

for clinicians who routinely perform continual professional development activities such as reading journal papers or online resources to keep up to date.

The traditional definition of evidence-based practice, provided by Sackett et al. (1996), has been questioned by Greenhalgh (2020) in light of the COVID-19 pandemic. Some pandemic-related interventions such as vaccines are amenable to population, intervention, comparator, outcome (**PICO**)-style research questions (discussed later in this chapter) and randomised controlled trials (see **Chapter 5: Experimental and Quasi-experimental Designs**); however, broader interventions such as social distancing, hand washing and the use of face coverings are more challenging to evaluate with the same rigour. This raises an important evidence-based practice question: should interventions with limited high-quality published data be delayed or ignored? Greenhalgh et al. (2020) argued for the 'precautionary principle', where acting without definitive evidence is sometimes warranted. In the definition above, Sackett et al. (1996) argued for the use of 'current best evidence', which frames a statement famously attributed to Maya Angelou:

> 'Do the best you can until you know better. Then when you know better, do better'

This statement captures the essence of evidence-based practice and is worth remembering.

How Prehospital Research Has Advanced

In the last 20 years, prehospital research has advanced significantly. In 2006, the UK national ambulance research steering group (NARSG) was founded, and chaired by Professor Niroshan Siriwardena (until 2018). NARSG aimed to unite UK ambulance services with the goal of facilitating prehospital research by helping researchers develop projects that are suitable and appropriate for ambulance services.

Several high-profile clinical trials have been successfully conducted within the prehospital setting internationally; see **Table 1.1**. Please note that **Table 1.1** is not exhaustive and is for illustrative purposes only.

There are also many notable clinical trials currently in progress, including: PATCH-Trauma in Australia, New Zealand and Germany assessing tranexamic acid in trauma (Mitra et al., 2021), RESIST in Denmark assessing remote ischaemic conditioning in stroke (Blauenfeldt et al., 2020) and EXACT in Australia assessing oxygen titration in out-of-hospital cardiac arrest (Bray et al., 2019), to name but a few.

In addition to the advance of clinical trials within the prehospital setting, large multiorganisational programmes of research have taken place, including programmes such as PhOEBE (Turner et al., 2019). Qualitative and mixed methods studies are also becoming more prevalent in prehospital research (McManamny et al., 2014).

Table 1.1 – Notable prehospital clinical trials.

Acronym	Title	Country
-	Intravenous drug administration during out-of-hospital cardiac arrest: A randomized trial (Olasveengen et al., 2009)	Norway
RSI	Prehospital rapid sequence intubation improves functional outcome for patients with severe traumatic brain injury: A randomized controlled trial (Bernard et al., 2010)	Australia
PACA	Effect of adrenaline on survival in out-of-hospital cardiac arrest: A randomised double-blind placebo-controlled trial (Jacobs et al., 2011)	Australia
RICH	Induction of prehospital therapeutic hypothermia after resuscitation from nonventricular fibrillation cardiac arrest (Bernard et al., 2012)	Australia
STREAM	Fibrinolysis or primary PCI in ST-segment elevation myocardial infarction (Armstrong et al., 2013)	International: 15 countries
LINC	Mechanical chest compressions and simultaneous defibrillation vs conventional cardiopulmonary resuscitation in out-of-hospital cardiac arrest: The LINC randomized trial (Rubertsson et al., 2014)	European: 3 countries
AVOID	Air versus oxygen in ST-segment-elevation myocardial infarction (Stub et al., 2015)	Australia
PARAMEDIC	Mechanical versus manual chest compression for out-of-hospital cardiac arrest (PARAMEDIC): A pragmatic, cluster randomised controlled trial (Perkins et al., 2015)	UK
FAST-MAG	Prehospital use of magnesium sulfate as neuroprotection in acute stroke (Saver et al., 2015)	USA
RINSE	Induction of therapeutic hypothermia during out-of-hospital cardiac arrest using a rapid infusion of cold saline: The RINSE trial (Rapid Infusion of Cold Normal Saline) (Bernard et al., 2016)	Australia

(continued)

Table 1.1 – Notable prehospital clinical trials. (*continued*)

Acronym	Title	Country
SAFER 2	Support and Assessment for Fall Emergency Referrals (SAFER) 2: A cluster randomised trial and systematic review of clinical effectiveness and cost-effectiveness of new protocols for emergency ambulance paramedics to assess older people following a fall with referral to community-based care when appropriate (Snooks et al., 2017)	UK
PARAMEDIC2	A randomized trial of epinephrine in out-of-hospital cardiac arrest (Perkins et al., 2018)	UK
AIRWAYS-2	Effect of a strategy of a supraglottic airway device vs tracheal intubation during out-of-hospital cardiac arrest on functional outcome: The AIRWAYS-2 randomized clinical trial (Benger et al., 2018)	UK
PART	Effect of a strategy of initial laryngeal tube insertion vs endotracheal intubation on 72-hour survival in adults with out-of-hospital cardiac arrest: A randomized clinical trial (Wang et al., 2018)	USA
RIGHT-2	Prehospital transdermal glyceryl trinitrate in patients with ultra-acute presumed stroke (RIGHT-2): An ambulance-based, randomised, sham-controlled, blinded, phase 3 trial (Bath et al., 2019)	UK
PRINCESS	Effect of trans-nasal evaporative intra-arrest cooling on functional neurologic outcome in out-of-hospital cardiac arrest: The PRINCESS randomized clinical trial (Nordberg et al., 2019)	European: 7 countries
PASTA	Effect of an enhanced paramedic acute stroke treatment assessment on thrombolysis delivery during emergency stroke care: A cluster randomized clinical trial (Price et al., 2020)	UK
CPAP	Prehospital continuous positive airway pressure (CPAP) for acute respiratory distress: A randomised controlled trial (Finn et al., 2021)	Australia

Service Evaluation, Clinical Audit and Quality Improvement

Service Evaluation

Service evaluation is a type of study that is considered to be different from research. The aim is to define or judge current care without reference to a standard (Health Research Authority, 2017). It asks the question 'what standard does this service achieve?'. This is different from **clinical audit** where a standard of care is set and the service is measured against the standard (discussed in the next section).

Service evaluation is not considered research because it does not aim to generate new generalisable or transferable knowledge using scientifically sound methods (Health Research Authority, 2021) and therefore does not require research ethics committee review (Health Research Authority, 2017). It is a useful approach to adopt when developing a new research project idea where evidence is limited or when current quality of care is unknown.

Service Evaluation Example

Pilbery et al. (2019) performed a service evaluation to determine how paediatric pain was assessed and managed by ambulance clinicians in a large region in England. Anonymised, routinely-collected clinical record data were utilised, which did not require research ethics committee review (Health Research Authority, 2017). It was found that 91% of children suffering moderate to severe pain achieved effective pain management (defined as a pain score reduction of ≥2 out of 10), although 87% of these did not receive analgesics. It was concluded that further research was needed to explain the significant rates of effective pain management in the absence of analgesic administration.

Clinical Audit

Clinical audit is an integral part of clinical governance that seeks to evaluate quality of care by measuring specific criteria against an agreed standard and then implementing a change to bring about improvement. Clinical audit is different from research. It is an ongoing process led by service providers that uses current knowledge, whereas research is often a one-off event led by researchers that generates new knowledge (Gottwald and Lansdown, 2014). Clinical audit asks the question 'are we doing the right thing in the right way?', whereas research asks 'what is the right thing to do?' (Gottwald and Lansdown, 2014).

Clinical audit involves measuring and improving quality of care over time against well-defined standards (Esposito and Dal Canton, 2014). Quality of care can be measured against documented interventions or observations, such as administering an analgesic for patients suffering severe pain or documenting a reason why an analgesic has not been administered, such as patient refusal or contraindication. Most ambulance services have several high-priority clinical audits for conditions such as cardiac arrest, heart attack and stroke, among others.

The PhOEBE project (Turner et al., 2019), a four-year mixed methods research project, recommended new ways of measuring quality in ambulance services, including:

- Mean change in pain score
- Proportion of serious emergency conditions correctly identified at the time of the 999 call
- Response time
- Proportion of decisions to leave a patient at scene that were potentially inappropriate
- Proportion of patients transported to the emergency department by 999 emergency ambulance who did not require treatment or investigation(s)
- Proportion of ambulance patients with a serious emergency condition who survive to admission, and to seven days post admission.

These measures or criteria of quality were deemed important by key stakeholders, including ambulance services, patients, the public, emergency care clinical academics, commissioners and policy makers. If ambulance services are not auditing these already, it is likely that they will be in the future.

Although clinical audit is not research, they are closely linked; research can inform clinical audit and vice versa. As mentioned above, the PhOEBE project (a research study) has made recommendations for criteria for clinical audit. This is because research asks 'what is the right thing to do?'. It turns out that reducing pain is one of the most important 'right things to do', as found by Turner et al. (2019). This has led to recommendations for clinical audit using mean pain score reduction as a criterion of quality.

Clinical audit can also inform research. If quality of care is monitored over time, and is found to decline over time, or during certain periods of time, this may prompt a research study to explore reasons for the change. Clinical audit is an important and valuable evidence-based practice tool that should be utilised to its full potential to ensure patients receive optimum care.

Quality Improvement
Quality improvement is defined as:

> 'the combined and unceasing efforts of everyone – healthcare professionals, patients and their families, researchers, payers, planners and educators – to make the changes that will lead to better patient outcomes (health), better system performance (care) and better professional development'
>
> (Batalden and Davidoff, 2007).

Whilst there is a clear distinction between clinical audit and research, the same cannot be said for quality improvement and research as there are areas of overlap between the two. Quality improvement is discussed comprehensively in **Chapter 10: Quality Improvement**.

The Research Process

The process of research generally follows eight broad steps, illustrated in **Figure 1.3**. These steps start from identifying a problem such as a gap in the evidence, a clinical problem encountered in practice or a system problem with the ambulance service, and end with the dissemination of research findings. These eight steps are discussed individually.

Identify a Problem

The first step in the research process is to identify a problem. This could be through making observations in clinical practice, witnessing a decline in quality of care through audit or identifying a gap in the evidence.

Making such observations and asking questions is the starting point in the scientific method; see **Figure 1.4**. Research in the prehospital setting often involves humans and therefore is considered a social science. Prehospital research is a science; hence, we are scientists. Within the UK, paramedics study for a BSc (Hons) Paramedic Science to gain registration. The type of degree, a *Bachelor of Science*, along with the title, paramedic *science*, emphasises that clinicians are also scientists. Therefore, good prehospital research follows the scientific method, illustrated in **Figure 1.4**, which adopts a method of falsification rather than verification. It is much easier to falsify a hypothesis than to verify one. Take the black swan analogy: a researcher

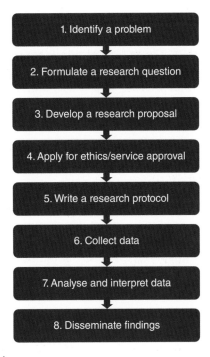

Figure 1.3 — The research process.

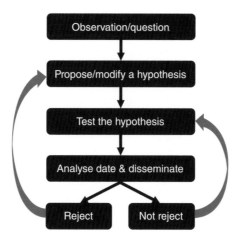

Figure 1.4 – The scientific method.
Source: Adapted from Law and Pascoe (2013).

may spend their whole life observing white swans and create a hypothesis that all swans are white. It has taken a significant amount of time to generate this hypothesis. However, if another researcher observes just one black swan on one day, the first researcher's lifetime of work is instantly disproved. The hypothesis would then be changed to 'all swans are white or black'. Hence, it is easier to disprove than prove a hypothesis.

An example of the scientific method at play in healthcare research is the association between smoking and lung cancer. Scientists (researchers and/or clinicians) observed in clinical practice that many people who develop lung cancer are smokers. A hypothesis was generated: 'smoking causes lung cancer'. This hypothesis was tested within the British Doctor's Study, a large **cohort study** (Doll and Hill, 1956; Doll et al., 2004). An association between smoking and lung cancer was observed; therefore, the hypothesis that lung cancer causes smoking was not disproved.

Once an observation has been made or a problem has been identified, an answerable research question should be formulated.

Formulate a Research Question

Developing an answerable research question might seem simple but it is one of the most challenging aspects of the research process. The entire research project is built on the foundation of the research question, so do not underestimate how much time and effort this step takes. The research question will likely go through several iterations before it is finalised.

Formulation of the research question is described in **Chapter 3: Systematic Reviews** as part of developing a systematic review question. The process is essentially the same and involves the use of a framework to structure the question. Common

a) PICO framework

Does intranasal fentanyl reduce pain score in children suffering pre-hospital acute pain more than oral paracetamol?

| Population | Intervention | Comparator | Outcome |

b) PICo framework

Why do paramedics have a fear of attending unwell children in the prehospital setting?

| Population | Phenomena of interest | Context |

Figure 1.5 – Worked research question examples using PICO and PICo.

frameworks include PICO (Population, Intervention, Comparator and Outcome), qualitative **PICo** (Population, phenomena of Interest and Context), **SPIDER** (Sample, Phenomenon of Interest, Design, Evaluation, Research type) and **SPICE** (Setting, Perspective, Intervention, Comparison and Evaluation). There are a significant number of research question frameworks available to assist in research question development – no fewer than 38 (Booth et al., 2019). Only a small number have been covered in this section. Please refer to the Booth et al. (2019) supplementary file for a comprehensive list of research question frameworks.

The PICO framework lends itself more to quantitative analysis, either through observational methods as discussed in **Chapter 4: Observational Studies** or through experimental methods as described in **Chapter 5: Experimental and Quasi-experimental Designs**. The qualitative PICo framework lends itself to qualitative methods, as discussed in **Chapter 6: Qualitative Research**.

Examples of formulating a research question using the PICO and qualitative PICo frameworks are shown in **Figure 1.5**.

Develop a Research Proposal

Once a research question has been created, the next step is to develop a research **proposal** (not a **protocol**). At this stage, it is a good idea to *involve the research department* of the service(s)/organisation(s) where you intend to conduct the study. They will support the development of the proposal, supply an early indication regarding the feasibility of the study and provide expertise. A research proposal should include the following sections as a minimum:

- **Research title**
  - This should be concise, clear and self-explanatory.
- **Research team**
  - All members of the proposed research team should be listed.

- **Background**

    - This provides context of the problem or question and answers the 'so what?' question. If someone asks 'so what?' or 'why is this important?', the background section of the proposal should be able to answer this. This section may include statistics on the scale of the problem or details of findings from previously published studies.

- **Research question and objectives**

    - The research question developed in the previous section should be included, along with any specific objectives.

- **Methods**

    - At this stage, the details of the methods do not have to be exhaustive, but a broad indication of study design, the population and data collection techniques should be provided as a minimum. Consider how research data will be stored and analysed.

- **Ethical considerations**

    - State whether ethical approval will be needed for the study. If unsure, speak to your local research department.

- **PPIE involvement**

    - PPIE is important in research and, where practical, efforts to involve patients and the public should be made. It should be stated in the proposal if PPIE is planned and if not, why it is not.

Funding

Before we move onto the next section, it would be useful to briefly discuss funding. Funding has not been included in **Figure 1.3** because it is not essential for conducting research, as some research can be conducted without funding, particularly reviews and small **observational studies**.

If the proposed research is significant, it may require funding to cover salaries and research costs. It is at this stage, after the research proposal has been developed, that research funding would be sought. This could be in the form of an external research grant from government or charitable sources, a training award, an internal organisational award or part of a programme of study, such as an MSc or PhD. Due to the variation in funding possibilities, not only at the national level but at the international level, funding has not been discussed here in any detail. If funding is required to conduct a research project, seek advice from your local research department.

Apply for Ethical/Service Approval

After the research proposal has been developed and funding has been considered and sought (if necessary), the next step is to apply for ethical (if necessary) and service/organisational (also termed research and development) approval. If you have involved the service/organisation research department from an early stage, as described in the 'develop a research proposal' section, gaining formal service/organisation approval should be a straightforward process. Problems may occur when a project has not been developed in collaboration with the research department, or without their knowledge, so early involvement is key.

Gaining ethical approval is a little more complex and may require the assistance of a more experienced researcher. Research projects that require ethical approval will need to state who the 'sponsor' is, in other words, which individual, organisation or partnership carries overall responsibility for the study. This might be an academic institution or an ambulance service.

Ethical approval can be gained from a university but in some cases it may be required at a broader level. For example, in England, if a research project involves National Health Service (NHS) patients, then NHS research ethics committee (REC) approval will be required, and will often form part of the overall Health Research Authority (HRA) application. Please refer to **Chapter 2: Ethics of Prehospital Research**, where the importance of ethics in prehospital research is discussed.

Write a Research Protocol

A research protocol is a full description of the study, and it should act as a 'manual' for researchers to follow, like a recipe book for baking a cake. It should be able to answer any question that arises during the whole research process, such as 'how should this data be analysed?', 'what should I do about missing data?', 'what should I do if a serious incident occurs?' and 'what is the primary outcome measure?'.

The protocol should be extremely comprehensive and cover all foreseeable components of the research project. The protocol provides transparency and, when published, acts as a point of reference so that people reading the research can determine if the researchers did what they said they were going to do. It should include all details of the study, including but not limited to: study design, population, data collection, data analysis, ethics and study procedures. Protocols for systematic reviews are discussed in **Chapter 3: Systematic Reviews** and protocols for experimental studies are discussed in **Chapter 5: Experimental and Quasi-experimental Designs**. Examples of a prehospital clinical trial and systematic review protocol are the AIRWAYS-2 clinical trial protocol (Taylor et al., 2016) and a systematic review protocol looking at medication errors in the prehospital paramedic environment (Walker et al., 2019).

All good researchers should pre-plan what they are looking for and what they wish to assess. There must be a strong foundation, a justification for why the researchers are looking at a specific outcome measure or association. This is because false associations can easily be found in routine data. If researchers analyse a dataset without an aim or objective, they are likely to find associations. Such associations may be unreliable, as '**confounding** by indication' may be present. An example of this is the association between ibuprofen and chickenpox in children. Munro (2019) argued that the evidence for ibuprofen causing children with chickenpox to become more unwell was tenuous and largely observational. In essence, children who are well with chickenpox do not need many medications and may, for example, only receive paracetamol if needed. Children who are more unwell with chickenpox tend to receive more medications, in this case paracetamol *and* ibuprofen. From an observational point of view, studies have concluded that children with chickenpox become more unwell when they receive ibuprofen. Munro (2019) argued for the opposite: more unwell children tend to require more medication, and children who are more unwell with chickenpox would still be more unwell, with or without ibuprofen. This 'confounding by indication' is important to remember, as *association does not equal causation*. The takeaway message is that if you analyse a dataset without a plan or purpose, you will probably find associations, but those associations may be confounded and misleading.

Collect Data

After developing and finalising a comprehensive research protocol, data collection can begin. Within the study protocol, information regarding type of data to be collected and where the data will be stored should have already been determined.

For a qualitative study, as discussed in **Chapter 6: Qualitative Research**, data might be audio/video recordings, field notes, photographs or documents. For a quantitative study, as discussed in **Chapter 4: Observational Studies** and **Chapter 5: Experimental and Quasi-experimental Designs**, or a consensus study, as discussed in **Chapter 8: Consensus Methods**, numerical data are collected, either from routine clinical data or a custom data collection tool, such as for a clinical trial or for a survey. If performing a mixed methods study, as discussed in **Chapter 7: Mixed Methods Research**, then often a mixture of numerical and non-numerical data are collected. If performing a systematic review, as discussed in **Chapter 3: Systematic Reviews**, then either numerical data, non-numerical data or a mixture of both, depending on the nature of the review, are collected from previously published studies.

Analyse and Interpret Data

Developing an answerable research question was described earlier as one of the hardest phases of the research process. The analysis and interpretation phase is arguably just as challenging, particularly when qualitative, non-numerical data are involved.

When dealing with numerical data, the statistical analysis is normally pre-determined, for reasons discussed in the 'write a research proposal' section. This makes the analysis reasonably straightforward. The interpretation can be more challenging, as it is very easy to overestimate findings and make ambitious recommendations for sweeping reform. At the start of this chapter, we stated: 'it is better to be uncertain than overconfident'. When interpreting quantitative findings and making recommendations for clinical practice and future research, it would be wise to remember this statement.

Non-numerical data are much more challenging to analyse. Imagine you performed 16 audio-recorded interviews with members of staff, each lasting around an hour.

After collecting the recordings, the data require transcription to translate them from audio format to written text format. The art of transcription is a challenge in itself. The result will be 16 documents of written text, each approximately 10,000 words in length. That is a total of approximately 160,000 words of data to analyse. Qualitative data analysis will not be discussed in any depth here; see **Chapter 6: Qualitative Research** for further guidance on this.

People often say that qualitative studies are easier to perform than quantitative studies. In our opinion, this is not true; they are both challenging in their own way, and qualitative data analysis is no mean feat.

Disseminate Findings

The final stage of the research process is the dissemination of findings. It could be argued that there is a further step that revolves around implementation science and implementing research findings into clinical practice. This was not described as a separate process as there is crossover here with quality improvement. One of the aims of quality improvement is to take current best evidence, adapt it to suit the local context and evaluate the effectiveness of the improvement initiative; quality improvement is described extensively in **Chapter 10: Quality Improvement**.

Effective dissemination is extremely important. Considering the time, effort and resources required to complete a research study from start to finish, as described in this chapter, imagine doing all that work and then failing to disseminate the findings effectively. No one would be aware of your work because they are not able to find it and therefore it cannot be implemented into clinical practice. At the start of this chapter, we defined research as 'increasing the stock of knowledge'. Without effective dissemination, research would not be added to the stock of knowledge, negating the main reason for doing research in the first place. Effective dissemination of research findings is paramount.

There are several strategies used to disseminate research findings, including:

- Publication in peer-reviewed journals
  - There are many peer-reviewed journals that accept prehospital research, including paramedicine and emergency medicine journals, along with major medical journals for studies with significant impact potential.
  - Writing a research report for publication is discussed in **Chapter 9: Critically Appraising a Paper and Preparing a Paper for Publication**.
- Presentation at conferences
  - There are a growing number of prehospital research conferences. These are not only great for presenting research findings, but also for networking and keeping up to date with the latest research.
- Video/animation/infographics
  - Increasingly, researchers are using various digital mediums to disseminate their findings, including recorded video or animated

presentations that can be posted to online video hosting websites and infographics that can be uploaded to websites or social media accounts.

- Executive summaries
  - An executive summary of the research findings can be developed and sent to key stakeholders, including policy and guideline makers, key organisations such as professional colleges or groups and individual ambulance services.

The Future

Most of the chief investigators for the studies shown in **Table 1.1** were medical doctors. There are a growing number of prehospital clinical academics internationally who are undertaking or have completed a doctorate in the field of paramedicine. As of 5 August 2021, there were 201 doctorates in the field of paramedicine registered on the **Paramedic PhD** website, including clinical (n = 185) and non-clinical (n = 16) researchers from the UK (n = 58), Australia (n = 58), the US (n = 22), Canada (n = 15) and South Africa (n = 10) (Paramedic PhD, 2021a). Considering the increase in clinical and non-clinical academics completing their doctorates in the field of paramedicine over the last 20 years (see **Figure 1.6**), it is likely that more prehospital research will be led by prehospital clinicians in the future.

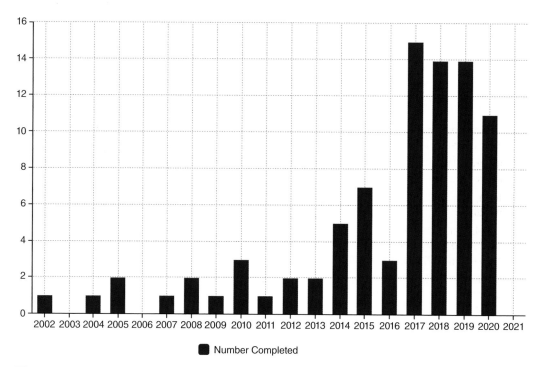

Number Completed

Figure 1.6 – Number of doctorates in the field of paramedicine completed by year.
Source: Paramedic PhD (2021b). Used with permission.

Clinical academics add value to research as they have a wealth of clinical experience coupled with academic skills, enabling them to explore possible solutions to everyday clinical problems. They have practical, pragmatic insights into routine clinical practice and are well placed to offer solutions when developing complex research projects. Trusson et al. (2019) concluded that clinical academics had the potential to provide significant benefit to research endeavours, but they should be encouraged and supported with ongoing post-doctoral scope to utilise their unique skills and experience, otherwise their value may not be recognised.

Summary

In this chapter, we have defined research and explained its importance for prehospital and paramedic practice, discussed theory and evidence-based practice, outlined the advances in prehospital research, described clinical audit and quality improvement, explained the research process from an initial idea to dissemination and highlighted areas for future development. We hope that this chapter provides a useful context and frames the rest of the textbook. We also hope that it and subsequent chapters will inspire you to get more involved in prehospital research. For the professionalisation of ambulance services and ambulance service staff, it is imperative that we build the prehospital evidence base and foster clinical academics. This will lead to higher quality research, higher quality care and, ultimately, improved patient outcomes.

References

Alderson, P. 1998. The importance of theories in health care. *BMJ (Clinical Research Ed.)*, 317, 1007–1010.

Ambulance Service of New South Wales. 2018. History. Available at: http://www.ambulance.nsw.gov .au/about-us/history.html [Accessed 10 July 2018].

Armstrong, P. W. et al. 2013. Fibrinolysis or primary PCI in ST-segment elevation myocardial infarction. *New England Journal of Medicine*, 368, 1379–1387.

Batalden, P. B. and Davidoff, F. 2007. What is 'quality improvement' and how can it transform healthcare? *Quality and Safety in Health Care*, 16, 2–3.

Bath, P. M. et al. 2019. Prehospital transdermal glyceryl trinitrate in patients with ultra-acute presumed stroke (RIGHT-2): An ambulance-based, randomised, sham-controlled, blinded, phase 3 trial. *The Lancet*, 393, 1009–1020.

Benger, J. R. et al. 2018. Effect of a strategy of a supraglottic airway device vs tracheal intubation during out-of-hospital cardiac arrest on functional outcome: The AIRWAYS-2 randomized clinical trial. *JAMA*, 320, 779–791.

Bernard, S. A. et al. 2010. Prehospital rapid sequence intubation improves functional outcome for patients with severe traumatic brain injury: A randomized controlled trial. *Annals of Surgery*, 252, 959–965.

Bernard, S. A. et al. 2012. Induction of prehospital therapeutic hypothermia after resuscitation from nonventricular fibrillation cardiac arrest. *Critical Care Medicine*, 40, 747–753.

Bernard, S. A. et al. 2016. Induction of therapeutic hypothermia during out-of-hospital cardiac arrest using a rapid infusion of cold saline: The Rinse trial (Rapid Infusion of cold Normal Saline). *Circulation*, 134, 797–805.

Bhaskar, R. 1975. *A Realist Theory of Science*, Routledge, Oxfordshire.

Blauenfeldt, R. A. et al. 2020. A multicentre, randomised, sham-controlled trial on REmote iSchemic conditioning In patients with acute STroke (RESIST) – Rationale and study design. *European Stroke Journal*, 5, 94–101.

Booth, A. et al. 2019. Formulating questions to explore complex interventions within qualitative evidence synthesis. *BMJ Global Health*, 4, E001107.

Bray, J. E. et al. 2019. The EXACT protocol: A multi-centre, single-blind, randomised, parallel-group, controlled trial to determine whether early oxygen titration improves survival to hospital discharge in adult OHCA patients. *Resuscitation*, 139, 208–213.

Caroline, N. L. 2007. *Nancy Caroline's Emergency Care in the Streets*, Jones and Bartlett Learning, Llc, Massachusetts.

Chamberlain, D. 2018. Looking back 70 years at the evolution of the paramedic. *Journal of Paramedic Practice*, 10, 282–283.

Ciottone, G. R. 2006. *Disaster Medicine*, Mosby Elsevier, Missouri.

Coster, J. et al. 2019. Outcomes for patients who contact the emergency ambulance service and are not transported to the emergency department: A data linkage study. *Prehospital Emergency Care*, 23, 566–577.

Creswell, J. W. 2014. *A Concise Introduction to Mixed Methods Research*, Sage Publications, California.

Davidoff, F. et al. 2015. Demystifying theory and its use in improvement. *BMJ Quality & Safety*, 24, 228–238.

Doll, R. and Hill, A. B. 1956. Lung cancer and other causes of death in relation to smoking; A second report on the mortality of british doctors. *British Medical Journal*, 2, 1071–1081.

Doll, R. et al. 2004. Mortality in relation to smoking: 50 years' observations on male british doctors. *BMJ*, 328, 1519.

Esposito, P. and Dal Canton, A. 2014. Clinical audit, a valuable tool to improve quality of care: General methodology and applications in nephrology. *World Journal of Nephrology*, 3, 249–255.

Finn, J. C. et al. 2021. Prehospital Continuous Positive Airway Pressure (CPAP) for acute respiratory distress: A randomised controlled trial. *Emergency Medicine Journal*, Epub ahead of print.

Gottwald, M. and Lansdown, G. 2014. *Ebook: Clinical Governance: Improving the Quality of Healthcare for Patients and Service Users*, Maidenhead, McGraw-Hill Education.

Green, H. E. 2014. Use of theoretical and conceptual frameworks in qualitative research. *Nurse Researcher*, 21.

Green, J. and Thorogood, N. 2018. *Qualitative Methods for Health Research*, Sage Publications, California.

Greenhalgh, T. 2020. Will Covid-19 be evidence-based medicine's nemesis? *Plos Medicine*, 17, E1003266.

Greenhalgh, T. et al. 2020. Face masks for the public during the Covid-19 crisis. *BMJ*, 369, M1435.

Guba, E. G. and Lincoln, Y. S. 1994. Competing paradigms in qualitative research. *In:* Denzin, N. K. and Lincoln, Y. S. (Eds.) *Handbook of Qualitative Research.* Thousand Oaks, CA: Sage.

Health Research Authority. 2017. Defining research table. Available at: http://www.hra-decisiontools.org.uk/research/docs/definingresearchtable_oct2017-1.pdf [Accessed 10 May 2021].

Health Research Authority. 2021. UK policy framework for health and social care research. Available at: https://www.hra.nhs.uk/planning-and-improving-research/policies-standards-legislation/uk-policy-framework-health-social-care-research/uk-policy-framework-health-and-social-care-research/ [Accessed 10 May 2021].

Jacobs, I. G. et al. 2011. Effect of adrenaline on survival in out-of-hospital cardiac arrest: A randomised double-blind placebo-controlled trial. *Resuscitation*, 82, 1138–1143.

Landhuis, E. 2016. Scientific literature: Information overload. *Nature*, 535, 457–458.

Law, G. R. and Pascoe, S. W. 2013. *Statistical Epidemiology*, CABI, Oxfordshire.

Lederman, N. G. and Lederman, J. S. 2015. What is a theoretical framework? A practical answer. *Journal of Science Teacher Education*, 26, 593–597.

Mcmanamny, T. et al. 2014. Mixed methods and its application in prehospital research: A systematic review. *Journal of Mixed Methods Research*, 9, 214–231.

Mitra, B. et al. 2021. Protocol for a multicentre prehospital randomised controlled trial investigating tranexamic acid in severe trauma: The PATCH-Trauma trial. *BMJ Open*, 11, E046522.

Moher, D. et al. 2009. Preferred reporting items for systematic reviews and meta-analyses: The PRISMA statement. *BMJ*, 339, B2535.

Munro, A. 2019. Varicella and NSAIDs – Are you too chicken to prescribe? [Accessed 21 April 2021]. Available at: https://doi.org/10.31440/DFTB.18763

Newton, A. 2012. The ambulance service: The past, present and future. *Journal Of Paramedic Practice*, 4, 303–305.

Nordberg, P. et al. 2019. Effect of trans-nasal evaporative intra-arrest cooling on functional neurologic outcome in out-of-hospital cardiac arrest: The Princess randomized clinical trial. *JAMA*, 321, 1677–1685.

OECD. 2015. Frascati manual 2015: Guidelines for collecting and reporting data on research and experimental development, the measurement of scientific, technological and innovation activities. Available at: http://dx.doi.org/10.1787/9789264239012-en [Accessed 18 April 2021].

Olasveengen, T. M. et al. 2009. Intravenous drug administration during out-of-hospital cardiac arrest: A randomized trial. *JAMA*, 302, 2222–2229.

Ontario Paramedic Association. 2015. History of paramedics in Ontario. Available at: https://www.ontarioparamedic.ca/before-9-1-1/history-of-paramedics-in-ontario [Accessed 10 July 2018].

Paramedic Phd. 2021a. Doctorate register. Available at: https://www.paramedicphd.com/registers/doctorate-register [Accessed 05 August 2021].

Paramedic Phd. 2021b. Statistics. Available at: https://www.paramedicphd.com/resources/statistics [Accessed 20 April 2021].

Perkins, G. D. et al. 2015. Mechanical versus manual chest compression for out-of-hospital cardiac arrest (PARAMEDIC): A pragmatic, cluster randomised controlled trial. *The Lancet*, 385, 947–955.

Perkins, G. D. et al. 2018. A randomized trial of epinephrine in out-of-hospital cardiac arrest. *New England Journal of Medicine*, 379, 711–721.

Phillips, D. C., Phillips, D. C. and Burbules, N. C. 2000. *Postpositivism and Educational Research*, Rowman and Littlefield, Maryland.

Pilbery, R., Miles, J. and Bell, F. 2019. A service evaluation of paediatric pain management in an English ambulance service. *British Paramedic Journal*, 4, 37–45.

Popper, K. R. 1962. *Conjectures and Refutation. The Growth of Scientific Knowledge*, New York, Basic Books.

Price, C. I. et al. 2020. Effect of an enhanced paramedic acute stroke treatment assessment on thrombolysis delivery during emergency stroke care: A cluster randomized clinical trial. *JAMA Neurology*, 77, 840–848.

Queensland Ambulance Service. 2018. QAS history and heritage. Available at: https://www .ambulance.qld.gov.au/history.html [Accessed 10 July 2018].

Rubertsson, S. et al. 2014. Mechanical chest compressions and simultaneous defibrillation vs conventional cardiopulmonary resuscitation in out-of-hospital cardiac arrest: The LINC randomized trial. *JAMA*, 311, 53–61.

Sackett, D. L. et al. 1996. Evidence based medicine: What it is and what it isn't. *BMJ*, 312, 71–72.

Saver, J. L. et al. 2015. Prehospital use of magnesium sulfate as neuroprotection in acute stroke. *New England Journal of Medicine*, 372, 528–536.

Schulz, K. F., Altman, D. G. and Moher, D. 2010. CONSORT 2010 statement: Updated guidelines for reporting parallel group randomised trials. *BMJ*, 340, C332.

Snooks, H. A. et al. 2017. Support and Assessment for Fall Emergency Referrals (SAFER) 2: A cluster randomised trial and systematic review of clinical effectiveness and cost-effectiveness of new protocols for emergency ambulance paramedics to assess older people following a fall with referral to community-based care when appropriate. *Health Technology Assessment*, 21.

Stub, D. et al. 2015. Air versus oxygen in ST-segment-elevation myocardial infarction. *Circulation*, 131, 2143–2150.

Sundstrøm, T. et al. 2014. Prehospital use of cervical collars in trauma patients: A critical review. *Journal of Neurotrauma*, 31, 531–540.

Tashakkori, A. and Teddlie, C. 2010. *Sage Handbook of Mixed Methods in Social and Behavioral Research*, Sage Publications, California.

Taylor, J. et al. 2016. Design and implementation of the AIRWAYS-2 trial: A multi-centre cluster randomised controlled trial of the clinical and cost effectiveness of the i-gel supraglottic airway device versus tracheal intubation in the initial airway management of out of hospital cardiac arrest. *Resuscitation*, 109, 25–32.

The Pleasure of Finding Things Out. 1981. [TV]. *Horizon*. BBC. Available at: https://www.bbc.co.uk/ iplayer/episode/p018dvyg/horizon-19811982-the-pleasure-of-finding-things-out [Accessed 18 April 2021].

Trusson, D., Rowley, E. and Bramley, L. 2019. A mixed-methods study of challenges and benefits of clinical academic careers for nurses, midwives and allied health professionals. *BMJ Open*, 9, E030595.

Turner, J. et al. 2019. Developing new ways of measuring the quality and impact of ambulance service care: The PhOEBE mixed-methods research programme. Programme Grants Appl Res. 7(3)

Voorberg, W. H., Bekkers, V. J. J. M. and Tummers, L. G. 2015. A systematic review of co-creation and co-production: Embarking on the social innovation journey. *Public Management Review*, 17, 1333–1357.

Walker, D. et al. 2019. Contributing factors that influence medication errors in the prehospital paramedic environment: A mixed-method systematic review protocol. *BMJ Open*, 9, E034094.

Wang, H. E. et al. 2018. Effect of a strategy of initial laryngeal tube insertion vs endotracheal intubation on 72-hour survival in adults with out-of-hospital cardiac arrest: A randomized clinical trial. *JAMA*, 320, 769–778.

Weaver, K. and Olson, J. K. 2006. Understanding paradigms used for nursing research. *Journal of Advanced Nursing*, 53, 459–469.

White, N. M. et al. 1973. Mobile coronary care provided by ambulance personnel. *British Medical Journal*, 3, 618–622.

Chapter 2

Ethics of Prehospital Research

Adèle Langlois, Steph Armstrong and Aloysius Niroshan Siriwardena

---

Chapter Objectives

This chapter will cover:

- Key ethical concepts in prehospital and emergency research
- UK and international ethical regulatory frameworks
- Types and models of consent in prehospital studies
- Ethical considerations and processes for front-line staff, managers and organisations involved and how these can be addressed
- Examples of studies involving prehospital consent

Introduction

This chapter considers and explores the key ethical considerations when undertaking prehospital research, the barriers to traditional models of consent, alternative approaches that have been developed and how these have been applied to processes for those involved in conducting prehospital studies. The prehospital research environment is in its infancy compared to research in secondary care (hospital settings) and primary care (GP practices), partly due to the additional ethical and logistic barriers.

Much of the current preoccupation with the ethics of prehospital ambulance research concerns the conduct of trials, which has been a rapidly developing field with an increasing number and scale of studies. This reflects the need for early or novel interventions in time-critical conditions such as out-of-hospital cardiac arrest, myocardial infarction ('heart attack'), stroke and trauma or the need to evaluate emergency and urgent care pathways (which are being redesigned to provide safe care in the community under increasing pressures from rising demand for services).

Trials in ambulance settings pose particular challenges due to the urgency of conditions attended, the requirement to provide treatment and trial procedures outside healthcare facilities and the requirement for **informed consent** or an alternative to this in situations of limited time or impaired patient capacity. The ethical procedures used in recent major ambulance trials such as PARAMEDIC (Perkins et al., 2015), PARAMEDIC2 (Perkins et al., 2018), SAFER 1 (Snooks et al., 2014), SAFER 2 (Snooks et al., 2017), RIGHT-2 (RIGHT-2 Investigators, 2019) and AIRWAYS-2 (Benger et al., 2018) have increased our understanding of the practical application to ambulance trials of some of the concepts described below.

Ethical Concepts

While medical ethics can be traced back to the Hippocratic Oath, research ethics at the international level were first regulated through the **Nuremberg Code** of 1947, in response to the abusive human experiments perpetrated by the Nazi regime during the Second World War. The code enshrined the key bioethical principle of informed consent: a person taking part in research must agree to do so voluntarily, with sufficient knowledge and understanding of what will be involved (Fluss, 2004; Vollmann and Winau, 1996). These principles were further reinforced and developed by the World Medical Association in 1964 in the code of ethics guiding doctors in research: the Declaration of Helsinki (World Medical Association General Assembly, 1964).

The code also embodies what are known as the 'four principles' or 'Georgetown principles': respect for autonomy (the ability to decide for oneself), non-maleficence (not doing harm), beneficence (doing good) and justice (acting fairly) (Beauchamp and Childress, 2012). Derived by philosophers Tom Beauchamp and James Childress and first published in their 1979 seminal text, *Principles of Biomedical Ethics*, these principles provide a framework for normative deliberation that is widely used by both researchers and medical practitioners. All four are pertinent to the prehospital research context: autonomy is integral to the informed consent process, potential benefits and harms have to be weighed quickly in the acute emergency setting and patients should have equal opportunity to take part in research, whether or not they have capacity to consent.

Recently, the sufficiency of the principles to cover all aspects of biomedical ethics has been questioned (Hellsten, 2015; Padela et al., 2015). Bioethics scholars are exploring concepts such as vulnerability, trust and solidarity to see whether they might be incorporated into a more holistic ethical framework. Like the four principles, each of these concepts has resonance for prehospital research. Autonomy is closely linked with vulnerability: the less autonomy someone has, the more vulnerable they are deemed to be. The temptation is to exclude from research all those considered potentially vulnerable, to avoid being (or being seen as) exploitative. Yet, excluding those who lack capacity on these grounds can exacerbate injustice in terms of access both to opportunities to take part in research and to relevant research results. Thus, attempts to do no harm have had the opposite effect (Haugen, 2010; Straehle, 2016).

Trust has a symbiotic relationship with vulnerability: without vulnerability, there is no need for trust. Increasingly, trust-based consent is seen to be as valid as information-based consent, as patients base their decision on whether to participate in health research as much on their trust (or lack of it) in the researcher, as on the information they have received, thus exercising a form of relational rather than individual autonomy (Dove et al., 2017; Kongsholm and Kappel, 2017). This may have particular relevance in an emergency setting, where the time available to both provide information and build trust is scarce.

Solidarity can be defined as 'shared practices reflecting a collective commitment to carry "costs" (financial, social, emotional, or otherwise) to assist others' (Prainsack and Buyx, 2012). Some people may choose to exercise this solidarity by taking part in research for the benefit of others. Where potential participants lack capacity to make such a choice, the question of whether their inclusion in research can be justified is raised. Existing research ethics guidelines vary on whether or not those unable to give consent should only be **enrolled** in research that may be of direct benefit to them (Langlois et al., 2021).

Ethical Rules and Guidelines for Prehospital Research

Most countries have national legislation, regulations or guidelines outlining how ethical principles can and should be implemented in medical and other research. None of these addresses prehospital research specifically, but several contain detailed requirements or guidance for research in emergency situations and/or research with participants unable to consent. Importantly, the fifth and subsequent revisions of the Declaration of Helsinki have sought to address some of the specific ethical barriers to emergency research (Vanpee et al., 2004).

The United Kingdom and the European Union

In the UK, clinical trials of medicinal products are governed by the Medicines for Human Use (Clinical Trials) Regulations (2004). These implement European Directive 2001/20/EC (MRC). The Directive does not allow an incapacitated adult to be enrolled in a clinical trial without the consent of their legal representative, but in 2006 the UK made an exception to this provision to enable research in emergency situations where treatment must be administered urgently and it is not practical to get surrogate consent beforehand, provided these arrangements have been approved by an ethics committee (see the Medicines for Human Use (Clinical Trials) Amendment (No.2) Regulations (2006)).

Other EU member states have made similar exceptions (Lemaire, 2005). These were possible because a directive in EU law is implemented through the national laws of member states, leaving room for interpretation. All clinical trials with incapacitated patients conducted under the Clinical Trials Regulations must relate directly to their life-threatening or debilitating clinical condition and it must be expected that they will benefit from the trial. There must be a prospective benefit to the participant, and this should outweigh any risk (CT Regulations).

The Clinical Trials Directive was replaced in 2022 by Regulation 536/2014. A regulation is different from a directive in that EU member states must comply with the regulation directly, rather than through national laws. The Clinical Trials Regulation contains provisions that will allow emergency research without consent if certain conditions are met. The trial must be one that can only be conducted in emergency situations and must relate directly to the medical condition that means it is not possible to obtain prior informed consent from either the participant or their representative. It must have the potential to be of direct clinical benefit to the participant and must pose minimal risk in comparison to standard treatment. Finally, the investigator must certify that they are not aware of any previously expressed objections to enrolment by the participant, and consent from the participant and/or their representative must be sought as soon as possible (EU Regulation 2014). Whether or not this Regulation will apply in the UK will depend on the length of the UK's transition period.

Other types of research with incapacitated participants in the UK fall under the Adults with Incapacity (Scotland) Act (2000), the Mental Capacity Act (2005) in England and Wales and the Mental Capacity Act (Northern Ireland) 2016. The Mental Capacity Act (2005) requires that for a person to have the capacity or competence to provide informed consent, they should be able to understand, retain and weigh up the information provided in order to make a choice (Coats, 2006; Coats and Shakur, 2005).

The provisions for research with incapacitated participants and emergency research are different from those in the Clinical Trials Regulations (Coats, 2006; Coats and Shakur, 2005). In England, Wales and Northern Ireland, research with incapacitated patients must relate to the condition that has impaired their capacity, or its treatment. It must not be possible to do the research effectively without those lacking capacity. If there is the potential for benefit to the participant, the burden imposed on them must not be disproportionate to this benefit. Where there is no potential direct benefit, the research must be intended to provide knowledge on the causes, treatment or care of the impairing condition and the risks to the participant must be negligible.

In emergency situations, the need to consult with the participant's relative or carer can be waived where both treatment and enrolment are urgent, but the researcher must obtain the agreement of an independent medical practitioner or, if there is not time to do this, ensure they comply with the **protocol** approved by the ethics committee who reviewed the project (MRC 2007). It is not possible to conduct research with incapacitated adults in Scotland without surrogate consent, except that which falls under the Clinical Trials Regulations (Scotland Act; MRC 2007).

Other States

The most comprehensive national regulations on emergency research are the 'Exception from Informed Consent' (EFIC) and 'Waiver of Informed Consent' (WIC) regulations adopted by the US in 1996. As well as setting out requirements around the purpose of the research, input from legal representatives and/or family members once available, and acceptable benefits and risks, these regulations stipulate that there must have been (a) prior consultation with representatives of the communities where the research will be conducted and from which participants will be drawn and

(b) public disclosure in these communities of the planned research and its expected benefits and risks (EFIC/WIC).

Australia and South Africa also have notable national policies. The Australian Tri-Council Policy Statement on Ethical Conduct for Research Involving Humans (2018) contains an 'Application' section for each of its articles, including that on research in individual medical emergencies. This explains that because participants in emergency research are vulnerable due to their incapacity, their welfare should be subject to special ethical protections, such as consultation with former and prospective participants and gaining consent in advance of the emergency situation if the latter can be identified (Australia 2018). In South Africa, under the Guidelines for Good Practice in the Conduct of Clinical Trials with Human Participants (2006), emergency care research is only permissible if it will be minimally invasive. Among other requirements, researchers must try to find out the religious and cultural sensitivities of incapacitated emergency care patients (South Africa 2006).

Enrolling Participants in Research Studies

Arguably the principal ethical consideration for research concerns the method by which participants are prospectively identified and enrolled in a study. There are several ways in which a participant can be enrolled, which are often dependent on the research method (for example, qualitative study, clinical trial), the condition being studied (for example, stroke, cardiac arrest, diabetes) and the type of intervention being trialled (for example, drugs trial, device trial, care pathways) (Armstrong et al., 2017). Where possible, it is considered best practice to enrol participants who have given informed consent; however, in the prehospital setting this may not be possible primarily as a result of reduced or impaired capacity.

Identification of Patients for Studies

For clinical trials, patients are recruited prospectively based on the inclusion and exclusion criteria for the study. This can also be the case for qualitative interview and **ethnographic** studies, although this can sometimes mean observations begin before consent is taken (Booker et al., 2019).

Other methods used in qualitative studies of patients who have contacted the ambulance include recruitment of people who have agreed to participate following previous studies or via charities and social media (McKinlay et al., 2020). Another method of recruitment for qualitative studies is to contact patients who have been recorded by the ambulance service after being attended with a specific condition (e.g. fracture, heart attack, stroke), ideally after checking with their general practitioner whether they are well enough and have the **mental capacity** to be interviewed (Iqbal et al., 2013; Togher et al., 2013, 2015).

Identification of patients for observational (cross-sectional, cohort, case-control) studies usually involves searching routine ambulance datasets (Coster et al., 2019; Siriwardena et al., 2019; Whitley et al., 2021).

Recruiting ambulance clinicians to studies, whether by invitation through their organisations, via identification by searching routine data or through social media, also needs careful consideration to ensure that ethical principles of confidentiality and informed consent are adhered to.

Whichever method is selected for identifying patients or practitioners, researchers need to comply with national and international legislation and organisational requirements on protection of data, such as the Data Protection Act 2018, the General Data Protection Regulations (Mondschein and Monda, 2019; Spencer and Patel, 2019) or the Caldicott Principles for information governance (Taylor, 2013).

Assessing Capacity

As we have seen, capacity is assessed as the ability to understand, retain and weigh up information and to additionally be able to communicate the desire to take part in research. The need to be able to assess capacity quickly whilst adhering to these principles is an important consideration in prehospital research. One suggested method is to follow a structured questioning process as follows (Appleton et al., 2017):

- Explain the condition and intervention to the participant.

- Ask the participant to repeat this information in their own words using targeted questions (understanding and retention) such as 'what do we think is wrong with you?', 'what are we going to do to treat you?' and 'what are we expecting to happen?'.

- Ask the participant if they have any further questions (weighing up).

- Ask the participant if they wish to take part in the research (communication of wishes).

If at any point the participant is not able to answer a question or if there are concerns regarding their comprehension, capacity should not be assumed, and an appropriate alternative method of enrolment should be explored.

The following section will identify different methods for enrolling participants in research studies, both for those that have capacity and those for whom capacity may be impaired.

Informed Consent

Informed consent relies on the assumption that the person giving it has the capacity to do so and that they have received enough information to make an informed decision. Often informed consent will include written consent, where the participant will complete and sign a consent form. The term 'written consent' can be used interchangeably with 'informed consent'; however, for consent to be given it does not need to be written. Oral informed consent may be used where the person giving consent is illiterate or has a physical impairment that prevents them from signing the form. For research purposes, the person taking the consent will usually record that oral consent has been given, by completing the form on behalf of the participant.

Exception From or Waived Consent

Prehospital research will often include some of the most acutely unwell patients, or patients who are distressed, making it difficult to gain informed consent due to impaired capacity (Armstrong et al., 2019). In these cases, research ethics committees can approve the use of exception from consent, where participants can be enrolled on the research study and given an intervention without giving consent because it is in their best interest to take part. For this method of enrolment to be valid, the participants should not have capacity to consent and there should be no viable alternative pool of participants. For example, research of interventions for cardiac arrest would not be possible in a conscious participant, who is not experiencing a cardiac arrest. In most cases where this type of enrolment method is used, participants are asked to confirm their consent retrospectively so that their data can be used once capacity has been regained, and some publications will refer to this as delayed consent (Armstrong et al., 2017). Participants may also be asked to consent to follow-up data collection once recovered from the initial incident.

Proxy or Surrogate Consent

In cases where the patient does not have capacity, consent may be gained from a surrogate or proxy. Surrogates can be a relative or close friend (partner), who will be asked to give their opinion as to whether the patient would have consented to take part if they had capacity to do so. Where there is no relative present and due to the timeliness of the intervention it would not be possible to identify such a person, a professional or legal surrogate can be used. In the hospital setting, this would be a named person who is not involved in any aspect of the study, who will assess the patient's suitability based on the inclusion criteria of the study and their immediate medical notes (Armstrong et al., 2019). They will then make a best-interest decision on behalf of the patient. In the prehospital setting, the short amount of time that the paramedic is in contact with the patient can make adoption of the professional surrogate role difficult. It could also be argued that a paramedic may not be independent of the trial because any paramedic at a scene would be involved in the patient's care (Armstrong et al., 2019). Where a paramedic signs the consent form on behalf of the patient, it has been suggested that rather than providing surrogate consent, the paramedic instead signs to confirm that the patient meets the inclusion criteria to become a participant in the trial, thereby not providing true surrogate consent (Armstrong et al., 2019). This would essentially be a documented form of **waived consent** and could trigger the process for later delayed consent when the participant regains capacity.

Short Consent/Assent

Short (or brief) consent, which could also be referred to as assent, could also be an alternative in prehospital settings where timeliness of intervention or transportation to hospital is paramount. This involves briefly explaining the intervention to the participant and asking them to indicate their agreement to receiving the intervention as part of the research project (Armstrong et al., 2017, 2019). The participant will then be contacted at hospital or shortly after the incident once the initial emergency has passed and asked to give informed consent to remain in the study, including use of data already collected and subsequent collection of follow-up data. This allows the participant to maintain autonomy, whilst minimising any potential delay in treatment. It also means that individuals who agreed to the intervention as part of their treatment can decide not to take part in the research.

Withdrawal of Consent

At all times, participants in research must have the right to withdraw from the study. Withdrawal of consent can happen at any time during data collection, and it is important to have processes in place to allow for this. Participants may request that personal identifying information about them (such as name, address, phone number) be removed from any files and databases. Where research results and non-personal data are anonymised, it may not be possible to remove these items retrospectively. If this is not possible due to anonymity of data, then this should be made clear to the participant during the enrolment and consent process.

Ethical Considerations for Services and Staff

Whilst enrolment of participants and the related consent processes are a primary ethical consideration in prehospital research, there are other ethical considerations that those involved in research must be aware of. Most jurisdictions require all research-active individuals to undertake **Good Clinical Practice** (GCP) training. GCP guidelines are a set of internationally recognised ethical and scientific-quality requirements produced by the International Conference on Harmonisation of Technical Requirements for Registration of Pharmaceuticals for Human Use (ICH). These requirements must be followed when designing, conducting, recording and reporting clinical trials or studies. In particular, the GCP guidelines set out the roles and responsibilities of the investigator, sponsor and research ethics committee in ensuring that the research is ethical and safe. GCP determines how and by whom adverse effects are reported; these can include serious and unexpected adverse effects. It is important that anyone involved in research understands GCP requirements prior to taking part.

GCP training is often a requirement of research ethics committee approval and some research funding bodies and clinical trials units. It should be undertaken by all members of the research team, especially those involved in enrolling and consenting participants and delivering the intervention. Training is increasingly being offered via online or e-learning platforms, and there are several GCP training providers worldwide ensuring that the training is tailored to the relevant legislation for the country in which the research is being done. The training itself takes about four hours to complete and the advantage of e-learning is that it can be completed in bite-sized chunks at a place and time that is convenient to the participant. This can be particularly useful for clinicians who work shift patterns. Face-to-face training courses are also available, and for some these are the preferred way of learning, not least because they offer the opportunity to ask questions and seek clarification.

Most trials will also have trial-specific training for those that are delivering the intervention. This training will also be delivered in a number of ways, although (as with GCP training) it is increasingly being delivered via online/e-learning platforms. This may involve watching videos and then completing a short assessment to ensure that the learning has been completed and understood. In some cases, face-to-face learning may be required as the clinicians need to practise using the intervention; this is particularly the case for interventions involving medical devices (Benger et al., 2018). When delivering trial-specific training to paramedics, it is important to ensure that they have access to the intervention/trial packs prior to enrolling their first patient. Even where training is delivered online, it is important to ensure that participating paramedics are shown the trial packs and paperwork they will use in the field.

Examples of Different Approaches to Consent

In the following examples, we provide details of brief and full informed consent taken by paramedics (**Box 2.1**), waiver and deferred consent (**Box 2.2**) and finally retrospective consent (**Box 2.3**) for recruitment to a prehospital clinical trial.

Box 2.1 Paramedic Consent

In the RIGHT **feasibility** trial of a transdermal glyceryl trinitrate patch for stroke (Ankolekar et al., 2012, 2013), potential participants with suspected stroke were approached by trained research paramedics to take part in the study. The paramedic explained the study to the patient by reading out a single-page information sheet on the purpose of the study, the reasons why they were approaching the patient and what would happen to them if they took part. To assess capacity to give consent, the paramedic asked simple questions about the information just provided to see if the patient had understood the trial, including 'what is your diagnosis?' (answer: stroke), 'what is wrong with your blood pressure?' (answer: it is high) and 'what is the treatment?' (answer: a patch). If the patient could answer correctly and agreed to take part in the study, they were asked to sign a consent form.

If the patient lacked capacity, their relatives if present were approached to provide consent on their behalf, termed proxy consent. If there was no relative present, research paramedics gave proxy consent on their behalf, provided that a second paramedic or ambulance technician was present and able to act as a witness to consent and countersign the form. The initial consent, from patient, relative or paramedic, covered the period in the ambulance up to and including admission to hospital.

Once the patient arrived in hospital, the hospital researcher discussed the trial again, provided a full patient information sheet and answered any questions. If the patient was unable to write, witnessed verbal consent was recorded on the

(continued)

Box 2.1 Paramedic Consent (*continued*)

consent form. If the patient lacked capacity (for example, in cases of dysphasia, confusion or reduced conscious level), proxy consent was sought from a relative. Full-informed, written consent was sought from each patient within 24 hours of initial consent and before the next treatment dose. If consent was not obtained within 24 hours, the trial intervention was withheld but blood pressure readings were taken until consent was obtained.

In contrast, the main RIGHT-2 trial (RIGHT-2 Investigators, 2019) enabled paramedics to complete written informed consent that covered the whole trial for patients with capacity. For those patients without capacity, proxy consent was obtained from an accompanying relative, carer or friend, if present, or from the paramedic if no accompanying person was present (as happened in the RIGHT feasibility study). Confirmatory consent was obtained from the patient, or their relative, carer or friend (if available), in hospital when the patient lacked capacity in the ambulance.

Although paramedics were successful in recruiting and consenting patients in the feasibility and main studies, they identified difficulties with the informed consent process as the greatest obstacle to enrolment, particularly when there were conflicting demands to care for the patient or respond to relatives' questions (Ankolekar et al., 2014).

Box 2.2 Waiver and Deferred Consent

In the PARAMEDIC2 trial of adrenaline in cardiac arrest (Perkins et al., 2018), written informed consent was deferred and sought from the patient when they had recovered and had been transferred to a hospital ward or discharged home. If they lacked capacity, consent was sought from a personal or professional legal representative.

The patient or legal representative was approached and provided with an information sheet explaining the trial, given time to consider the information provided and offered an opportunity for a study team member to return later to discuss participation further and take consent if this was agreed. The patient or legal representative could decide it was not an appropriate time to discuss the trial or they could decide not to take part, in which case their feelings were respected and their decision about taking part was recorded.

General information about the trial and sources of further information were made available throughout the trial via ambulance and university trial websites, newsletters, posters and information leaflets shared with GP practices, pharmacies, emergency departments and waiting areas. The trial team also developed a system to allow people to refuse in advance to take part in the trial in the event of a cardiac arrest by completing an online form or contacting the team by telephone or email, whereupon they were posted a stainless steel 'No Study' bracelet and, with their permission, their home address was passed to the ambulance service to register their wishes. Those requesting a 'No Study' bracelet were also told to tell those close to them of their wishes and that these wishes would be respected by the treating paramedics. Paramedics were trained to look for the bracelet.

Box 2.3 Retrospective Consent

In the SAFER 2 trial of paramedic assessment and referral, where appropriate, of older adults after a fall to a community falls pathway (Snooks et al., 2012, 2017), retrospective consent to follow-up was sought rather than brief or full consent or waiver. This was deemed acceptable because potential participants may have been in distress and so unable to give informed consent. Participants were contacted first by post, and then if needed by telephone or home visit, to record informed consent. Anonymised follow-up through linked records was also used to gather **outcome** data for patients who could not be contacted or who did not respond to requests for consent.

Whilst these methods of consent were acceptable at the time, they should not automatically be deemed acceptable for future studies. Each study should undergo a thorough review and selection of the most appropriate model of consent. Prehospital research is still evolving and as our understanding of capacity and consent in this field increases, so does our ability to conduct ethically sound clinical research.

Summary

This chapter provides an overview of UK and international ethical principles and regulatory frameworks in prehospital and emergency research; explains the different approaches to consent in prehospital studies; describes the processes for staff and organisations involved in conducting trials and studies in an ambulance setting; and provides examples of recent studies which have used different approaches to consent.

Further Reading

The following studies, from the Network exploring Ethics of Ambulance Trials (NEAT), funded by the Wellcome Trust, summarise recent evidence on the ethics of ambulance trials.

Armstrong, S. et al. 2017. Assessment of consent models as an ethical consideration in the conduct of prehospital ambulance randomised controlled clinical trials: A systematic review. *BMC Medical Research Methodology*, 17, 142.

Armstrong, S. et al. 2019. Ethical considerations in prehospital ambulance based research: Qualitative interview study of expert informants. *BMC Med Ethics*, 20, 88.

Langlois, A., Armstrong, S. and Siriwardena, A. N. 2021. Do national and international ethics documents accord with the consent substitute model for emergency research? *Academic Emergency Medicine*. 28, 569–577.

References

Ankolekar, S. et al. 2012. Determining the feasibility of ambulance-based randomised controlled trials in patients with ultra-acute stroke: Study protocol for the "Rapid Intervention with Gtn in Hypertensive stroke Trial" (RIGHT, ISRCTN66434824). *Stroke Research and Treatment*, 2012, 385753.

Ankolekar, S. et al. 2013. Feasibility of an ambulance-based stroke trial, and safety of glyceryl trinitrate in ultra-acute stroke: The Rapid Intervention with Glyceryl trinitrate in Hypertensive stroke Trial (RIGHT, ISRCTN66434824). *Stroke*, 44, 3120–3128.

Ankolekar, S. et al. 2014. Views of paramedics on their role in an out-of-hospital ambulance-based trial in ultra-acute stroke: Qualitative data from the Rapid Intervention with Glyceryl trinitrate in Hypertensive stroke Trial (RIGHT). *Annals of Emergency Medicine*, 64, 640–648.

Appleton, J. P. et al. 2017. Ambulance-delivered transdermal glyceryl trinitrate versus sham for ultra-acute stroke: Rationale, design and protocol for the Rapid Intervention with Glyceryl trinitrate In Hypertensive stroke Trial-2 (RIGHT-2) trial (ISRCTN26986053). *International Journal of Stroke*, 1747493017724627.

Armstrong, S. et al. 2017. Assessment of consent models as an ethical consideration in the conduct of prehospital ambulance randomised controlled clinical trials: A systematic review. *BMC Medical Research Methodology*, 17, 142.

Armstrong, S. et al. 2019. Ethical considerations in prehospital ambulance based research: Qualitative interview study of expert informants. *BMC Medical Ethics*, 20, 88.

Beauchamp, T. L. and Childress, J. F. 2012. *Principles of Biomedical Ethics*. New York; Oxford, Oxford University Press.

Benger, J. R. et al. 2018. Effect of a strategy of a supraglottic airway device vs tracheal intubation during out-of-hospital cardiac arrest on functional outcome: The Airways-2 randomized clinical trial. *JAMA*, 320, 779–791.

Booker, M. J. et al. 2019. Ambulance use for 'primary care' problems: An ethnographic study of seeking and providing help in a UK ambulance service. *BMJ Open*, 9, E033037.

Coats, T. J. 2006. Consent for emergency care research: The Mental Capacity Act 2005. *Emergency Medicine Journal*, 23, 893–894.

Coats, T. J. and Shakur, H. 2005. Consent in emergency research: New regulations. *Emergency Medicine Journal*, 22, 683–685.

Coster, J. et al. 2019. Outcomes for patients who contact the emergency ambulance service and are not transported to the emergency department: A data linkage study. *Prehospital Emergency Care*, 23, 566–577.

Dove, E. S. et al. 2017. Beyond individualism: Is there a place for relational autonomy in clinical practice and research? *Clinical Ethics*, 12, 150–165.

Fluss, S. S. 2004. The evolution of research ethics: The current international configuration. *Journal of Law, Medicine and Ethics*, 32, 596–603.

Haugen, H. M. 2010. Inclusive and relevant language: The use of the concepts of autonomy, dignity and vulnerability in different contexts. *Medicine, Health Care and Philosophy*, 13, 203–213.

Hellsten, S. K. 2015. The role of philosophy in global bioethics: Introducing four trends. *Cambridge Quartlerly of Healthcare Ethics*, 24, 185–194.

Iqbal, M., Spaight, P. A. and Siriwardena, A. N. 2013. Patients' and emergency clinicians' perceptions of improving prehospital pain management: A qualitative study. *Emergency Medicine Journal*, 30, E18.

Kongsholm, N. C. H. and Kappel, K. 2017. Is consent based on trust morally inferior to consent based on information? *Bioethics*, 31, 432–442.

Langlois, A., Armstrong, S. and Siriwardena, A. N. 2021. Do national and international ethics documents accord with the consent substitute model for emergency research? *Academic Emergency Medicine*. 28, 569–577.

Lemaire, F. 2005. Waiving consent for emergency research. *European Journal of Clinical Investigation*, 35, 287–289.

Mckinlay, A. et al. 2020. Patient views on use of emergency and alternative care services for adult epilepsy: A qualitative study. *Seizure*, 80, 56–62.

Mondschein, C. F. and Monda, C. 2019. The EU'S General Data Protection Regulation (GDPR) in a research context. *In:* Kubben, P., Dumontier, M. and Dekker, A. (Eds.) *Fundamentals of Clinical Data Science*. Springer, New York.

Padela, A. I. et al. 2015. [Re]considering respect for persons in a globalizing world. *Developing World Bioethics*, 15, 98–106.

Perkins, G. D. et al. 2015. Mechanical versus manual chest compression for out-of-hospital cardiac arrest (PARAMEDIC): A pragmatic, cluster randomised controlled trial. *Lancet*, 385, 947–955.

Perkins, G. D. et al. 2018. A randomized trial of epinephrine in out-of-hospital cardiac arrest. *The New England Journal of Medicine*, 379, 711–721.

Prainsack, B. and Buyx, A. 2012. Solidarity in contemporary bioethics – Towards a new approach. *Bioethics*, 26, 343–350.

RIGHT-2 Investigators. 2019. Prehospital transdermal glyceryl trinitrate in patients with ultra-acute presumed stroke (RIGHT-2): An ambulance-based, randomised, sham-controlled, blinded, phase 3 trial. *Lancet*, 393, 1009–1020.

Siriwardena, A. N. et al. 2019. Patient and clinician factors associated with prehospital pain treatment and outcomes: Cross sectional study. *The American Journal of Emergency Medicine*, 37, 266–271.

Snooks, H. et al. 2012. Support and Assessment for Fall Emergency Referrals (SAFER 2) research protocol: Cluster randomised trial of the clinical and cost effectiveness of new protocols for emergency ambulance paramedics to assess and refer to appropriate community-based care. *BMJ Open*, 2.

Snooks, H. A. et al. 2014. Support and Assessment for Fall Emergency Referrals (SAFER 1): Cluster randomised trial of computerised clinical decision support for paramedics. *Plos One*, 9, E106436.

Snooks, H. A. et al. 2017. Paramedic assessment of older adults after falls, including community care referral pathway: Cluster randomized trial. *Annals of Emergency Medicine*, 70, 495–505.

Spencer, A. and Patel, S. 2019. Applying the Data Protection Act 2018 and general data protection regulation principles in healthcare settings. *Nursing Management (Harrow)*.

Straehle, C. 2016. Vulnerability, health agency and capability to health. *Bioethics*, 30, 34–40.

Taylor, P. 2013. Caldicott 2 and patient data. *BMJ*, 346, F2260.

Togher, F. J., Davy, Z. and Siriwardena, A. N. 2013. Patients' and ambulance service clinicians' experiences of prehospital care for acute myocardial infarction and stroke: A qualitative study. *Emergency Medicine Journal*, 30, 942–948.

Togher, F. J. et al. 2015. Reassurance as a key outcome valued by emergency ambulance service users: A qualitative interview study. *Health Expect*, 18, 2951–2961.

Vanpee, D., Gillet, J. B. and Dupuis, M. 2004. Clinical trials in an emergency setting: Implications From the fifth version of the Declaration of Helsinki. *Journal of Emergency Medicine*, 26, 127–131.

Vollmann, J. and Winau, R. 1996. Informed consent in human experimentation before the Nuremberg Code. *BMJ*, 313, 1445–1449.

Whitley, G. A. et al. 2021. The predictors, barriers and facilitators to effective management of acute pain in children by emergency medical services: A systematic mixed studies review. *Journal of Child Health Care*, 25, 481–503.

World Medical Association General Assembly. 1964. Human experimentation: Code of ethics of the World Medical Association (Declaration of Helsinki). *Canadian Medical Association Journal*, 91, 619.

Chapter 3

Systematic Reviews

Ffion Curtis, Despina Laparidou and Gregory Adam Whitley

Chapter Objectives

This chapter will cover:

- The definition of a systematic review
- Differentiation between different types of review
- The process and importance of developing and registering your systematic review protocol
- In-depth examination of the stages of a systematic review
- Developing and conducting your own systematic review

What is a Systematic Review?

A **systematic review** is defined as 'a review of the evidence on a clearly formulated question that uses systematic and explicit methods to identify, select and critically appraise relevant primary **research**, and to extract and analyse data from the studies that are included in the review' (Centre for Reviews and Dissemination, 2008).

Traditionally, systematic reviews were predominantly quantitative and often synthesised **randomised controlled trials** using techniques such as **meta-analysis**. In recent years, the number of systematic reviews of qualitative studies has increased, along with the number of systematic mixed studies reviews which include both types of research. Whichever type you are conducting, it is equally important to apply a systematic and explicit methodology (Aromataris and Munn, 2020).

Aim of a Systematic Review

There is an ever-increasing volume of health-related research articles being published. Systematic reviews aim to identify, evaluate, synthesise and summarise the findings from relevant individual studies, ensuring that the available evidence is more accessible to a wider audience (for example, researchers, healthcare professionals and decision makers).

A systematic review, when conducted well, will adhere to a strict scientific design based upon explicit, pre-specified and reproducible methods (Bridle, 2003). In addition to establishing what is known about a given topic, systematic reviews can also be used to identify gaps in the evidence base, which guide future research (Jones et al., 2017).

Different Types of Review

Before conducting your review, it is important to identify what type of review would best answer your research question, as there are several to consider. Here we provide a brief overview of some of the different review types.

Literature Review

Traditional literature reviews (also termed narrative reviews) can provide a summary of the evidence and are often influential. They do not employ the same explicit methodology in identifying, appraising and synthesising the research evidence as with the systematic review, and, as such, there is an increased likelihood of biased conclusions being drawn (Bridle, 2003).

Rapid Review

Rapid reviews are suitable when there is a need to provide information quickly to support decision making, often focused on new and emerging areas of research. They are defined as 'a form of knowledge synthesis that accelerates the process of conducting a traditional systematic review through streamlining or omitting specific methods to produce evidence for stakeholders in a resource-efficient manner' (Garritty et al., 2020).

Methodologies can vary, often omitting some of the lengthier (and more rigorous) processes of the standard systematic review. These reviews will often take less than six months to complete, depending on resources and the experience of the team, and they tend to present a narrative summary or a categorisation of retrieved evidence (Featherstone et al., 2015).

Scoping Review

Scoping reviews (or systematic scoping reviews) are useful for exploring the literature when very little is known about a topic and for answering a broader research question than a systematic review. It is still recommended that you adhere to the same rigorous methodological approach as when conducting a systematic review, and there is a **PRISMA** Extension for Scoping Reviews (PRISMA-ScR) to guide the conduct and reporting process (Tricco et al., 2018). This type of review is useful in identifying what evidence there is on a given topic, along with gaps in the literature. In some cases, a scoping review will lead to a more focused systematic review.

If your research question is more focused and you are interested in the effectiveness of an intervention or in learning about the experiences and perceptions of your population of interest, a systematic review will often be the best approach. From here on, we will focus our discussion on systematic review methodology.

The Review Team

It is important that you have the right people included within your review team. Ideally, a minimum of 2–3 reviewers will be involved in all key stages of the review process to reduce the potential for error and **bias** (Centre for Reviews and Dissemination, 2008). You should aim to involve several stakeholders who will be able to contribute a wide range of skills and expertise to your review, including clinical and topic experts, systematic reviewers and research methodology experts. In addition to this, you may wish to establish an advisory group whom you can consult at different stages of your review, which could include healthcare professionals, service users and patient representatives. Engaging with a wide range of stakeholders will help ensure that your review question has practical relevance in a real-world setting.

Developing a Systematic Review Research Question

Having identified a priority research topic, the first stage of performing a systematic review is to develop and refine your research question. To reduce the potential for bias, it is important that review questions are well-formulated, and that the methods used to answer them are specified a priori (before the study begins). You should begin by performing some scoping searches online to explore the existing literature in the area. This is an essential process to ensure that a systematic review on your topic has not already been done. If you find your review has already been conducted, you can explore if it needs updating or revise your review question and/or inclusion criteria. There are also systematic review **protocol** registration databases (such as **PROSPERO**, Database of Abstracts of Reviews of Effects (DARE)) that you can check to ensure that other review teams are not in the process of conducting your planned review (Centre for Reviews and Dissemination, 2008). If you do find that there is a planned review, this can be an opportunity to explore potential collaborations.

Defining the research question can take time, and it is critical that you formulate a clear, answerable research question. For example: 'what is the effect of a lifestyle intervention on type-2 diabetes?'. This question is too broad; how would you answer it? We don't know what the intervention is, what we are comparing it to or what the main **outcome** measure is.

If conducting a review of intervention studies, **PICO** (Population, Intervention, Comparator, Outcome) should be used as a framework for your research question (Harris et al., 2013). See **Box 3.1** for an example of a PICO research question.

There are several variations of framework acronyms available, the choice of which to use largely depends upon your research methodology. They include **SPIDER** (Sample, Phenomenon of Interest, Design, Evaluation, Research type) for qualitative and mixed methods approaches, **SPICE** (Setting, Perspective, Intervention, Comparison and Evaluation) and **PICo** (Population, phenomena of Interest and Context) for qualitative approaches. Your review question will provide the framework for protocol development and all subsequent stages of your review (inclusion/exclusion criteria and key search terms). Developing your review question and protocol will often be an iterative process and should include consultation with the relevant stakeholders.

Box 3.1 PICO Example Research Question

A description of the population:	**Population**	Adults with type-2 diabetes
An identified intervention:	**Intervention**	Physical activity
An explicit comparison:	**Comparison**	Metformin
Relevant outcomes:	**Outcome**	HbA1c (blood glucose)

Research question: What is the effect of a physical activity programme compared to metformin on HbA1c in adults with type-2 diabetes?

Protocol Development and Registration

Performing a systematic review is like baking a cake; you need a recipe to follow (the protocol), which will result in a tasty cake (the systematic review). If someone else were to pick up your recipe (protocol), they should be able to create the same cake (systematic review). This makes a systematic review reproducible, and therefore more reliable.

A systematic review protocol is the 'recipe' describing the key stages for the conduct of your systematic review. Here we present the key stages in conducting a systematic review, which includes the core elements of your systematic review protocol (see **Figure 3.1**).

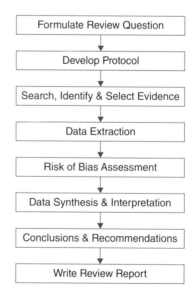

Figure 3.1 – Key stages in conducting a systematic review.

When developing your protocol, it is good practice to adhere to relevant reporting guidelines, such as the Preferred Reporting Items for Systematic reviews and Meta-Analyses (PRISMA) protocols (Moher et al., 2015). The guidelines can facilitate both protocol development and the final reporting of the systematic review. The protocol should include:

- A brief background on the topic you are investigating, including a strong justification for performing the systematic review.

- Review objectives and research question – you will need to determine the scope of your review, that is, the precise question to be asked.

- A search strategy – report the databases that you will search, including dates, terms and an example search strategy. State whether forward and backward citation tracking will be used, and describe methods for retrieving literature that is not obtainable via the usual publishing channels (grey literature such as reports, theses and conference proceedings) and ongoing studies (trial registers and contact with researchers in the field are useful sources).

- Inclusion criteria – this should be detailed, should be informed by components of the review question (such as PICO) and should explain the *process* (number of reviewers involved, whether the process will be independent and how disagreements between reviewers will be resolved).

- Data extraction – describe what data you plan to extract from the included studies, along with the *process*.

- **Critical appraisal** / quality assessment – specify criteria/checklist(s) to be used for appraising the methodological quality of included studies and the *process*.

- A method of synthesis – this may be to tabulate data and provide a **narrative synthesis**, or a meta-analysis (quantitative) or **meta-synthesis** (qualitative) (including details of the data analysis software you plan on using).

Additional considerations to include within your protocol include a project timeline, resources required (library resources, reviewers' time) and a dissemination plan.

Registration and/or publication of the review protocol is considered best practice and helps to avoid duplication of reviews, promotes transparency and reduces potential for bias (Stewart et al., 2012). There are various registration sites you may consider, such as OSF pre-registration or PROSPERO – the international database of prospectively registered systematic reviews in health and social care, welfare, public health, education, crime, justice and international development – where there is a health-related outcome (Centre for Reviews and Dissemination, 2020). It is important to consider your title; ideally it will contain your PICO and state that it is a systematic review. If known at this point, you should also include the type of analyses you intend to conduct (Moher et al., 2015).

Searching for Literature

It is critical to build an effective search strategy. This will be an iterative process informed by stakeholder consultation and preliminary searches to identify relevant terms. The review question and your inclusion/exclusion criteria will also inform your search strategy. Your aim is to create an extensive and reproducible search strategy (Bridle, 2003). Ideally an academic librarian or information specialist will support you in developing your search strategy and identifying appropriate databases, keywords and subject headings (such as Medical Subject Headings (MeSH)).

A search strategy should maintain a balance between sensitivity (identifying all relevant information/references) and specificity (excluding irrelevant information/references). Your search strategy, depending on the type of review you are conducting, will aim to locate mainly peer-reviewed journal articles, but possibly also books, conference abstracts and grey literature (that is, research and reports produced by organisations, businesses, industry and the government, which are not controlled by the traditional commercial or academic publishers) (Godin et al., 2015). Searching in bibliographic databases is the most efficient way to identify relevant studies. You should also supplement your searches with internet searches (that is, Google Scholar), as well as forward and backward citation tracking (that is, looking into the references and locating further relevant studies) from the included studies and review articles you have identified.

Contacting experts in the field and hand searching key journals and relevant systematic reviews will also help locate relevant studies. You may consider core and specialised bibliographic databases (such as MEDLINE, Embase and CINAHL Complete), depending on your review topic. Some of the most commonly used databases and search engines are: AMED (Allied and Complementary Medicine); ASSIA (Applied Social Science Index and Abstracts); British Nursing Index; CINAHL (Cumulative Index of Nursing and Allied Health Literature); Cochrane Central Register of Controlled Trials; Cochrane Database of Systematic Reviews (CDSR); Cochrane Library; Embase; King's Fund; MEDLINE; Ongoing trials registers; PsycINFO; and Web of Science. The number of databases you choose to search will depend upon your topic, as well as the time and resources you have available. For a comprehensive search, a minimum of two databases plus hand searching of selected journals is recommended (Suarez-Almazor et al., 2000). A comprehensive search strategy should consist of both relevant keywords and subject headings for each concept of your review question/topic. Search techniques include truncation, proximity operators and phrase searching, which you can then combine using **Boolean operators**; see **Box 3.2**.

All databases will have a help section describing their own search technique tools and how to operate. With this in mind, please be aware that you may need to 'translate' your search strategy for different databases. This means that whilst it still needs to be the same strategy, you may need to use different searching tools and amend some terms and subject headings. Also, when inputting your terms, remember

Box 3.2 Systematic Review Search Techniques

Truncation:

psycholog* will retrieve: psychology, psychologist, psychological.

Proximity searching:

Within operator; for example, eating W5 disorder finds the words if they are within *five words* of one another and *in the order in which you entered them.*

Near operator; for example, eating N8 disorder finds the words if they are within *eight words* of one another regardless of the order in which they appear.

Phrase searching:

Placing double quotation marks ("____") around two or more words ensures that only resources containing that exact phrase are found; for example "heart attack".

Boolean operators – AND/OR/NOT

OR broadens your search by retrieving results that include either of your terms:

anorexia nervosa **OR** bulimia.

AND narrows your search by retrieving results that include both of your terms:

anorexia nervosa **AND** antidepressants.

NOT refines your search, but use with care:

anorexia **NOT** bulimia.

that there may be alternative ways to describe concepts, such as alternative spellings (for example, behaviour in the UK and behavior in the US) or terms (caregiver and carer). You can also use subject headings or MeSH terms, depending on the database you are searching, to help you identify and include all terms that may fall under the term you are interested in.

You can also use search limiters, for example, to include only randomised controlled studies or to look for papers published during certain periods (such as between 2000 and 2015) or in certain languages. Unless you have a very strong reason for doing so (for example, a medication that went into circulation at a specific point in time), which should also be clearly documented, it is preferable to not put any limitations on your search strategies.

Before conducting your literature search, it is important to do some preliminary scoping searches to assess the volume of literature in your area, and to identify additional keywords, databases and other resources to search.

For an example of a search strategy, see **Table 3.1**.

Table 3.1 – Search strategy example.

	MEDLINE	CINAHL Complete	PsycINFO	Embase	Scopus	Web of Science Core Collection
S1	Infant* OR Child* OR Pediatric* OR Paediatric* OR Adolescen* OR (MH "Pediatrics") OR (MH "Adolescent")	Infant* OR Child* OR Pediatric* OR Paediatric* OR Adolescen* OR (MH "Pediatrics") OR (MH "Adolescence")	Infant* OR Child* OR Pediatric* OR Paediatric* OR Adolescen* OR DE "Pediatrics"	Infant* OR Child* OR Pediatric* OR Paediatric* OR Adolescen* OR Pediatrics/ OR adolescent/ OR child/	TITLE-ABS-KEY ((infant* OR child* OR pediatric* OR paediatric* OR adolescen*) AND (ambulance* OR "Emergency Medical Service*" OR prehospital OR pre-hospital OR "Out of hospital" OR paramedic*) AND (pain OR analgesi*))	TS = ((Infant* OR Child* OR Pediatric* OR Paediatric* OR Adolescen*) AND (Ambulance* OR "Emergency Medical Service*" OR Prehospital OR Pre-hospital OR "Out of hospital" OR Paramedic*) AND (Pain OR Analgesi*))
S2	Ambulance* OR "Emergency Medical Service*" OR Prehospital OR Pre-hospital OR "Out of hospital" OR Paramedic* OR (MH "Emergency Medical Services") OR (MH "Ambulances")	Ambulance* OR "Emergency Medical Service*" OR Prehospital OR Pre-hospital OR "Out of hospital" OR Paramedic* OR (MH "Emergency Medical Services") OR (MH "Ambulances")	Ambulance* OR "Emergency Medical Service*" OR Prehospital OR Pre-hospital OR "Out of hospital" OR Paramedic* OR DE "Emergency Services"	Ambulance* OR "Emergency Medical Service*" OR Prehospital OR Pre-hospital OR "Out of hospital" OR Paramedic* OR ambulance/		
S3	Pain OR Analgesi* OR (MH "Acute Pain") OR (MH "Pain Management")	Pain OR Analgesi* OR (MH "Pain") OR (MH "Pain Management")	Pain OR Analgesi* OR DE "Pain"	Pain OR Analgesi* OR Pain/ OR analgesia/		
S4	S1 AND S2 AND S3	S1 AND S2 AND S3	S1 AND S2 AND S3	S1 AND S2 AND S3		

Finally, remember that your search must be accurately documented and reproducible. Make sure to keep detailed records of the databases you searched, the number of articles you retrieved from each database, how many duplicates you excluded and how many articles you have for each step of the screening process (see sections below). Completing a PRISMA flow diagram is considered best practice (Moher et al., 2009).

Screening and Retrieving Literature

Having completed your searches, you will quite likely have a lengthy list of potentially relevant references, maybe tens, hundreds or even thousands. The next step is to export the reference lists from individual databases and combine them for screening to determine relevance for your review. There is often some overlap between the databases, so you may get some duplication in references retrieved. This is because journals generally index their publications in more than one database. It is important to accurately document the *total number of results* from your search before and after duplicates are removed. As you move through the screening process it is essential to document how many papers are removed at each stage. This will enable you to complete a PRISMA flow diagram (Moher et al., 2009). Please see **Figure 3.2** for an example of a PRISMA flow diagram.

To combine your reference list for screening, there are a range of reference manager software programmes available (for example, EndNote, Mendeley, Zotero), or alternatively this can be done in Microsoft Excel. Many databases (such as Ovid SP, EBSCOHost and Scopus) have a simple export function for search results, although some have a maximum number of titles and abstracts you can export at once; therefore, you may have to export your results in small 'bundles'. The help section within the individual databases will have instructions on how to do this. References retrieved from supplementary searches (Google Scholar, screening reference lists of included papers and some grey literature sources) may need to be added manually.

Remove Duplicates

Reference managers often have built-in duplicates recognition software to help you identify and remove duplicate papers. This will identify some duplications, but possibly not all. This is because software only works on exact matches and there can be variation in how the references are formatted (for example, lists of author names are not exactly the same, or the journal name is indexed as the short name). After the electronic removal of duplicates, you should manually screen the papers to identify and remove any remaining duplicates. If using Microsoft Excel, you will need to manually identify and remove all duplicates. It is useful to sort by title and to eyeball the papers as you scroll down, then sort by author and eyeball again. Once all duplicates have been removed, document the number of duplicates for your PRISMA flow diagram, and then move onto the title and abstract screen.

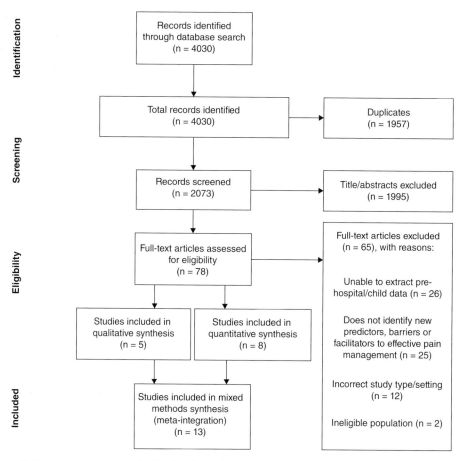

Figure 3.2 – Example of a PRISMA flow diagram.
Source: PRISMA flow diagram from Whitley et al. (2021).

Title and Abstract Screen

Ideally this stage should be completed independently by two reviewers, with any discrepancies resolved through discussion with a third reviewer (Harris et al., 2013). If this is not possible and only one reviewer screens the titles and abstracts, it is important to report this as a weakness when writing up your review, as the likeliness of missing important references will be higher. Due to the potentially large volume of references that require screening at the title and abstract stage, it needs to be as simple as possible. It is advisable to create a brief screening tool (checklist) based on the inclusion and exclusion criteria. You should also pilot the screening tool to ensure it is effective and that all review team members would reach the same decision when using it. The duration of this task will depend upon the number of references retrieved. It is important not to rush this activity, as you don't want to accidentally exclude relevant references.

Start by reading the title of each paper. If it is immediately apparent that the paper is not relevant, then it can be excluded. If for example you are looking specifically for studies involving adults and the title states '... in pre-term babies', you can confidently exclude the paper. If there is any doubt, or you feel the paper could be relevant, read the abstract. Having read the abstract, if you cannot confidently exclude the reference, you must include it for the next stage of screening: full-text screening (Centre for Reviews and Dissemination, 2008). At the end of this process, document the number of papers excluded from the title and abstract screen for your PRISMA flow diagram.

Full-text Retrieval

You should now have a significantly reduced number of references for which you will need to obtain full-text copies for a more detailed screening process. Whilst an increasing number of articles are Open Access, many require journal subscriptions. For those registered with a university, this step is relatively straightforward. Educational institutions will have subscriptions to a range of different journals, and for those papers you cannot access, it may be possible to request an interlibrary loan through your library service.

For those not registered at a university, accessing full-text journal articles may be less straightforward. There are many alternative options for retrieving full-text papers, including extending the review team or contacting corresponding authors and requesting full-text copies of articles. **Box 3.3** shows an email template to request a full-text paper.

Alternative methods for gaining full-text papers include utilising local initiatives; check with your local research department to see what services are available to you (for example, the Library and Knowledge Services (LKS) for NHS ambulance services in England).

Box 3.3 Email Template to Request a Full-text Paper From a Corresponding Author

Subject: Article request

Dear Dr Bill Lord,

My name is John Smith and I'm a paramedic working for the East Midlands Ambulance Service NHS Trust in the UK. I'm performing a systematic review looking at prehospital pain management in children and your paper titled 'Effects of the introduction of intranasal fentanyl on reduction of pain severity score in children: An interrupted time-series analysis' published in *Pediatric Emergency Care* appears to fit my inclusion criteria. Unfortunately, I'm unable to access the full-text paper.

Would you mind sending the above full-text PDF paper so that I can complete my systematic review? Thank you for your time taken to read this and I look forward to hearing from you.

Yours sincerely,

John.

Full-text Screen

Once you have all your full-text papers, you need to screen them carefully according to your inclusion and exclusion criteria. This will ideally be conducted independently by two reviewers, as it has been reported that one reviewer may miss up to 8% of eligible studies when screening alone (Centre for Reviews and Dissemination, 2008). Any discrepancies between two reviewers should be resolved through discussion or with the inclusion of a third reviewer. There are various study eligibility tools available that you may adapt for your review such as the Cochrane data extraction form, or alternatively create your own based upon your review PICO/inclusion criteria. It is a good idea to also pilot this tool on a few studies initially to ensure it is fit for purpose. It is useful to include details of the reviewer completing the task, date completed and location within the articles where data were sourced for eligibility. The number of exclusions and the reasons for exclusion will be included in your PRISMA flow diagram. See **Figure 3.2** for an example of a PRISMA flow diagram.

Having screened and retrieved all relevant papers, the next step is to extract relevant data and critically appraise each study that has met the eligibility criteria for your systematic review.

Data Extraction

Data extraction refers to the systematic recording and structured presentation of data from your included studies. In this context, data refers to any information about or from your included study and may include study authors, aims, methodology, participants, context, outcomes and findings (Bridle, 2003). A standardised data extraction provides consistency, improves validity and **reliability** and reduces potential bias (Centre for Reviews and Dissemination, 2008). There are many data extraction templates available, such as those provided by Cochrane and the Joanna Briggs Institute, to guide you in this process. A well-designed data extraction form should facilitate the conduct of your systematic review, including the risk of bias assessment, data syntheses and meta-analyses (Li et al., 2019).

When extracting data, it is important to strike the right balance between extracting too few or too many data. Too few data will result in having to go back to the original studies when you are conducting the syntheses and write-up; too many data would not be an efficient use of your time as a reviewer. The best approach is to find a suitable template and adapt it as necessary to suit your systematic review. When developing the data extraction form, you will need to consider your review question, the information that will be needed to conduct your review and how you will be presenting your data. An important part of this process will of course be piloting the form, testing how it works in practice. Ideally this will be performed by more than one reviewer, and for more than one study. A second reviewer should also check for accuracy by cross-checking forms with primary data sources (that is, included studies). Data extraction forms may be revised at this stage.

It is recommended that two reviewers independently extract data from all included studies to minimise risk of errors and the introduction of biases by review authors. However, where this is not feasible, it is acceptable for one reviewer to extract data, with a second reviewer cross-checking for accuracy (Buscemi et al., 2006).

Once you have collected your data, it is useful to present them in tabulated electronic format to provide a snapshot view of the included studies. This is useful as it enables the classification of studies for comparisons and subgroup analysis (Li et al., 2019). Also, this can be an opportunity to identify potential clinical or methodological heterogeneity or missing data (Bridle, 2003).

Critical Appraisal and Tools

In the context of a systematic review, quality assessment (critical appraisal) assesses **internal validity**, that is, the reliability of results based on the potential for bias. Bias refers to the extent to which the observed findings may be due to factors other than the named intervention/phenomena, and could be caused by inadequacies in the design, conduct or analysis of the primary studies (Harris et al., 2013).

Assessing the quality of the studies included in a systematic review is extremely important. For example, if you use high-quality ingredients when baking a cake, you are much more likely to create a high-quality cake (although the baker influences this process significantly!). The same is true for systematic reviews; the quality of the findings is reflected in part by the quality of the included studies (similarly, the researcher has a lot to do with this process). All the other steps in this chapter are important and they all contribute to the final quality of the systematic review, but if we look at critical appraisal in isolation, high-quality studies included in a systematic review will generally produce higher quality, more reliable results. Unfortunately, researchers have no control over the quality of the references retrieved in their systematic review; it is reliant entirely on the available literature. It is important to formally assess the quality of studies included in your systematic review against predefined criteria (Harris et al., 2013) and to consider the implications this may have on your final conclusions.

You can conduct the critical appraisal prior to data extraction, as you may decide to exclude studies that are deemed to be 'low quality' (Porritt et al., 2014). Alternatively, you can include low-quality studies and acknowledge the limitation within the review. If conducting a systematic review and meta-analysis of quantitative studies, you may include all studies that meet your inclusion criteria in the main analysis, and then conduct a sensitivity analysis (see Meta-analysis section in this chapter). This involves running additional meta-analyses with amended inclusion criteria based on quality rating (that is, removing the low-quality studies and reporting the effect this has on your results). Whichever option you choose, it is important that you describe your approach within your protocol a priori (Aromataris and Pearson, 2014) and are transparent in your reporting. The findings of your critical appraisal will often be informative for the future recommendations section of your systematic review.

Numerous critical appraisal scales and checklists have been developed. The most appropriate tool(s) for your review should be determined by your topic and, in particular, the design of the studies being appraised. Critical appraisal tools are often presented as a list of questions with examples given regarding how best to answer each question. See **Table 3.2** for examples of some of the tools that may be useful to you.

The list of tools in **Table 3.2** is by no means exhaustive and represents only a handful of the tools available to critically appraise research papers. Whichever tool you use, two reviewers should perform independent critical appraisal of included studies, with any disagreements resolved through discussion with a third reviewer (Aromataris and Munn, 2020). Once all included papers have been appraised using an appropriate tool, the findings should be presented in a table so that readers of the systematic review can scan *across* the included studies to get a feel for the overall risk of bias. Colours can be used to represent the risk of bias for each answer, generally red (high risk), amber (uncertain) and green (low risk), or ticks and crosses to illustrate whether a criterion has been satisfied or not. In some instances, it is also possible to calculate an overall study quality/bias rating. However, you may find it more informative to

Table 3.2 – Critical appraisal tools.

Source	Type of study
The Cochrane handbook https://training.cochrane.org/handbook	RCT, non-randomised experimental studies.
Joanna Briggs Institute (JBI) https://jbi.global/critical-appraisal-tools	RCT, non-randomised experimental studies, cohort, case control, case series, case report, analytic cross sectional, diagnostic, economic evaluation, prevalence, qualitative, opinion.
Critical Appraisal Skills Programme (**CASP**) https://casp-uk.net/casp-tools-checklists/	RCT, cohort, case control, diagnostic, economic evaluation, qualitative.
The mixed methods appraisal tool (MMAT) for systematic mixed studies reviews https://doi.org/10.1016/j.ijnurstu .2009.01.009	Quantitative, qualitative and mixed methods studies.

simply present ratings for each domain for readers to interpret alongside the review findings. An example of a critical appraisal table can be seen in **Table 3.3**.

In the example provided, you will see that risk of bias was low across many domains of these randomised controlled trials of cognitive behavioural therapy (CBT) interventions for insomnia in tinnitus patients. It was deemed high for blinding of participants and personnel, as it is almost impossible to blind individuals to behavioural interventions such as CBT (that is, both participants and personnel can tell who is receiving the intervention). There are also some domains where it is unclear as to whether there is the potential for bias; in this case it was due to poor reporting. Where there is missing information in articles, you can try and contact authors to ascertain risk of bias for different domains.

Once the critical appraisal is complete, the next stage of the systematic review is synthesis of the data.

Evidence Synthesis

The aim of synthesis within a systematic review is to produce more than the sum of its parts. This involves combining the results from primary studies to generate a whole (like a jigsaw puzzle); each study provides an individual jigsaw piece, whereas all the studies combined create a bigger picture. Sometimes the picture is clear, sometimes it

Table 3.3 – Critical appraisal table example.

	Risk of bias					
Study ID	Random sequence generation	Allocation concealment	Blinding of partici- pants and personnel	Blinding of outcome assessment	Incom- plete out- come data	Selective outcome reporting
Andersson 2005	Low	Unclear	High	Unclear	Low	Low
Beukes 2017	Low	Low	High	Low	Low	Low
Jasper 2014	Low	Low	High	Unclear	Low	Low
Kaldo 2007	Low	Low	High	Unclear	Unclear	Low
Weise 2016	Low	Low	High	Unclear	Low	Low

Source: Curtis et al. (2021).

is incomplete and messy. It is the role of the systematic review team to highlight what can be deduced from the evidence, what is missing and how the evidence base can move forward.

There are four major types of evidence synthesis: narrative synthesis, meta-analysis, meta-synthesis and **meta-integration**; see **Table 3.4**.

Narrative Synthesis

A **narrative synthesis** is a common approach to synthesising evidence within a systematic review and is defined as a non-numerical analysis of the overall findings. It should not be confused with the broader term 'narrative review', which is a non-systematic review. It is more subjective than a meta-analysis and, therefore, should be conducted with a rigorous and transparent approach to reduce the potential for risk of bias. Aspects of a narrative synthesis will often be included alongside other types of synthesis to provide context and support the interpretation of the collected evidence (Centre for Reviews and Dissemination, 2008). A narrative synthesis might be used when a meta-analysis cannot be performed, perhaps due

Table 3.4 – Types of synthesis.

	Type of synthesis			
	Narrative synthesis	**Meta-analysis**	**Meta-synthesis**	**Meta-integration**
Type of studies included in the review	**Quantitative.** When the included studies are very different (heterogenous). **Qualitative.** Only when a meta-synthesis is not possible. See Narrative synthesis section.	**Quantitative.** When the included studies are very similar (homogenous). See Meta-analysis section.	**Qualitative.** See Meta-synthesis section.	**Quantitative *and* Qualitative.** Used in systematic mixed studies reviews. See Meta-integration section.
Description	A non-numerical analysis of the overall findings within a systematic review.	A statistical technique for combining numerical data from multiple quantitative studies.	An integrative technique to combine non-numerical data from multiple qualitative studies.	A technique used to combine the findings from a quantitative *and* a qualitative synthesis.

to significant heterogeneity (Campbell et al., 2018). Where qualitative studies are included in a systematic review, a meta-synthesis should be considered (see Meta-synthesis section in this chapter).

This is an evolving area of work and there are guidelines for the development and conduct of narrative syntheses (Campbell et al., 2018; Popay et al., 2006).

The guidance framework consists of four elements:

- Developing a theory of how the intervention works, why and for whom
- Developing a preliminary synthesis of findings of included studies
- Exploring relationships within and between studies
- Assessing the robustness of the synthesis.

During the reporting of the results, individual study findings are often presented in a table, with the narrative synthesis findings reported in the text following the table.

One of the challenges in performing a narrative synthesis may be the volume of data, as many studies could be included in your systematic review and they may report on slightly different populations and contexts. It is easy to end up with a mass of data, a 'grey storm' of data if you like, that you struggle to make sense of. A solution to this is to generate themes to aid the discussion and provide clarity for the reader (and also for the researcher). For example, findings could be discussed in relation to their effectiveness and their safety, separately. Alternatively, an existing theoretical model could be used to help structure the analysis. For example, the biopsychosocial model of health (Engel, 1977) is often used in healthcare research and could be used in a narrative synthesis to frame the analysis. This would result in themes relating to the biological, psychological and social impact of the phenomenon being assessed. The use of this model would be termed using a 'framework', and if a framework is used it should be described within the methods. For example, 'a narrative synthesis was performed using the biopsychosocial model of health (Engel, 1977) as a framework'. Using an existing framework or developing your own framework by creating themes helps to provide structure to what could otherwise be a messy amalgamation of data that is difficult to make sense of. For further reading, see Centre for Reviews and Dissemination (2008) and Campbell et al. (2018).

Narrative Synthesis Example

Eaton et al. (2020) performed a study titled 'Contribution of paramedics in primary and urgent care: A systematic review'. A narrative synthesis was adopted and although an existing framework was not used, themes were generated to give structure to the analysis; therefore, the authors created their own framework. Six themes were created: description of the clinical role; clinical work environment; reduction in GP workload; patient satisfaction; clinical activities in primary care; and education and training. This provided a clear structure for the reader to focus on specific aspects and a clear view of these individual aspects *across* studies, generating a combined new view. This systematic review also compared the findings of the narrative synthesis with the existing literature.

Meta-analysis

If you are conducting a systematic review of quantitative studies, you will most likely want to conduct a statistical synthesis using a technique called meta-analysis. By combining the results of several studies, it is possible to provide a more reliable and precise estimate of an intervention's effectiveness than you would from one study alone. It is a powerful approach, combining outcomes from distinct, yet similar studies, with the potential to provide sufficient population numbers and generalisable population data to make more powerful evidence-based conclusions (Centre for Reviews and Dissemination, 2008).

Prior to conducting a meta-analysis, it is important to firstly determine if a statistical synthesis is appropriate, with consideration of your included studies and availability of data. In deciding this, you will need to firstly identify if there is any heterogeneity (variability) evident that would make it unwise to statistically combine your study data: are the studies that have met your systematic review eligibility criteria similar enough to combine within a meta-analysis? If there are differences between the participants, intervention characteristics or outcomes of included studies that could affect the pooled results of your analysis, they should not be combined this way. Studies should only be combined if they are similar enough to produce a meaningful average effect (Bridle, 2003).

It is recommended that you develop your 'characteristics of included studies' table to inform your decision-making processes at this stage. This will enable you to eyeball the data and identify any missing data or potential sources of clinical or methodological heterogeneity (Higgins et al., 2002). An example of a study characteristics table has been provided from Curtis et al. (2021); see **Table 3.5**.

In the example shown in **Table 3.5**, the Andersson study was included in the systematic review but *not* the meta-analysis. Whilst they did report a measure of

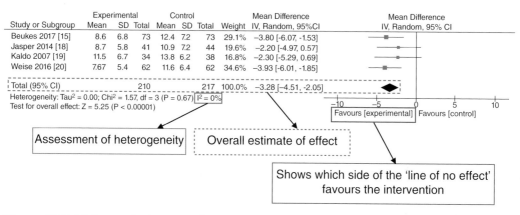

Figure 3.3 Meta-analysis example.
Source: Curtis et al. (2021).

Table 3.5 – Study characteristics table example.

Study (country)	Sample size	Intervention, frequency, duration and components	Comparison	Sleep outcome measure, end point, study finding
*Andersson et al., 2005 Sweden	Intervention: 12 Control: 11	CBT group sessions, 2 hours weekly for six weeks. Tinnitus information, applied relaxation (four sessions), cognitive restructuring, behavioural activation, positive imagery, sound enrichment using environmental sounds, exposure to tinnitus, hyperacusis advice, hearing tactics, relapse prevention and management of sleep	Waiting list control group	Sleep quality: visual analogue scale (0–100mm, anchors 'much pleased – 'not at all pleased'). Diary recordings over a week at 5 weeks. No significant interaction.
Beukes et al., 2017 United Kingdom	Intervention: 73 Control:73	Internet delivered audiologist guided CBT-based self-help, 2–3 modules released weekly over 8 weeks with weekly therapist contact via secured online messaging system. 16 recommended modules & 5 optional (including sleep module). Applied relaxation, thought analysis, cognitive restructuring, imagery and exposure techniques	Weekly monitoring control group	ISI, post intervention. Significant improvement in intervention compared to control (3.8±2.7)

(continued)

Table 3.5 – Study characteristics table example. (*continued*)

Study (country)	Sample size	Intervention, frequency, duration and components	Comparison	Sleep outcome measure, end point, study finding
Jasper et al., 2014 Germany	Intervention: 41 Control: 44	Internet delivered CBT-based self-help program, 12 mandatory and 6 optional text modules (including sleep module) and weekly therapist contact via a secured online messaging system. 10 week intervention. Applied relaxation, positive imagery, focus exercises, exposure to tinnitus, cognitive restructuring, and avoidance behaviour	Web-based discussion forum	ISI, post assessment. Pre-post Cohen's d (95% CI) 0.68 (0.22–1.14). Change score 2.3 (0.9–3.8)
Kaldo et al., 2007 Sweden	Intervention: 34 Control: 38	CBT-based self-help book guided by brief telephone support. 7 weekly phone calls over 6 weeks. Tinnitus information, defining goals, applied relaxation, positive imagery, focus exercises, exposure to tinnitus, sound enrichment, hyper sensitivity to sounds, hearing tactics, cognitive re-structuring, sleep management, concentration management, treatment summaries & evaluation, planning maintenance of positive effects and relapse prevention.	Wait-list control group	ISI, post treatment. Significant interaction favouring intervention effect [$F(1,69)=11.2$; $P<.002$]

Study (country)	Sample size	Intervention, frequency, duration and components	Comparison	Sleep outcome measure, end point, study finding
Weise et al., 2016 Sweden	Intervention: 62 Control: 62	Internet delivered audiologist guided CBT-based self-help program, 12 mandatory, and 6 optional modules and weekly therapist contact via a secured online messaging system. 10-week intervention. Applied relaxation, positive imagery, focus exercises, exposure to tinnitus, cognitive restructuring, sleep management and avoidance behaviour.	Online discussion forum	ISI, maximum of 4 weeks post treatment. Significant improvement in intervention compared to control. Hedges g(95%CI) 0.66 (0.30–1.02)

*not included in meta-analysis

Source: Curtis et al. (2021).

insomnia (the primary outcome), they did not use the same tool to measure the primary outcome of the review. If you decide that it is not appropriate to conduct a statistical synthesis, then you may conduct a narrative summary of included studies instead.

If at this stage it seems appropriate to conduct a meta-analysis, you will firstly need to calculate a measure of treatment effect with its 95% **confidence intervals** (CIs) for all individual studies. The summary statistics usually used to measure treatment effect include odds ratios (OR), relative risks (RR) and mean differences. A meta-analysis enables you to then combine the findings from two or more studies to calculate a weighted average of overall treatment effect (Akobeng, 2005). There are various packages to create your forest plot (meta-analysis); RevMan is commonly used as it is straightforward to use and free to download. **Figure 3.3** shows an example of a forest plot generated to estimate the average effect of cognitive behavioural therapy on insomnia in adults with tinnitus (Curtis et al., 2021).

The forest plot provides a visual representation of data from the individual studies, as well as an estimate of the overall point estimate. Again, you can eyeball the plot to visually assess if any heterogeneity is present (point estimates on different sides of the line of no effect, and CIs that do not overlap between some studies). The I^2 statistic, which is produced by default in the forest plot, will tell you whether statistical heterogeneity is present. The diamond shape represents the overall estimate of effect with confidence intervals. If this crosses the centre line (line of no effect), then the overall findings are non-significant. In this instance, it is clearly favouring the experimental group.

An example of how this forest plot would be reported: meta-analysis of four studies demonstrated a statistically significant between-groups difference in the Insomnia Severity Index score following CBT-based interventions (-3.28, 95% CI -4.51, -2.05, $P < 0.001$). There was no evidence of statistical heterogeneity, $I^2 = 0\%$. Whilst this is statistically significant, it is the role of the review team to interpret these findings and decide if they are clinically meaningful.

If you have studies with a high risk of bias, you can perform a sensitivity analysis to determine robustness of review findings by conducting additional analyses with the removal of some studies. Lower quality studies with a higher risk of bias are more likely to report inflated effect sizes. This could affect your findings and result in you incorrectly reporting a positive intervention effect. However, this isn't always the case and all studies that have met your inclusion criteria may provide important information, so a sensitivity analysis can form an important part of your statistical analysis. You may also wish to conduct sub-group analyses for the studies included in your systematic review, grouping on pre-defined criteria, such as population or intervention characteristics (Deeks et al., 2020). For example, if you are assessing the effectiveness of an intervention, you may wish to run separate analyses for interventions of different durations. Perhaps your intervention is effective if delivered for 12 weeks, but not for 8 weeks, for example.

Meta-synthesis

A meta-synthesis is the synthesis of qualitative data from studies included within your systematic review of qualitative and/or mixed methods studies that include a qualitative component. The purpose of a meta-synthesis (also known as a qualitative review or qualitative meta-synthesis) is to integrate and interpret findings from various similar qualitative studies that are exploring the same phenomena or experience (Ring et al., 2011). When developing and reporting a qualitative systematic review and meta-synthesis, it is best practice to follow well-established guidelines, such as the ENTREQ guidelines for enhancing transparency in reporting the synthesis of qualitative research (Tong et al., 2012).

You will need to familiarise yourself with the data by reading and re-reading the results sections of your included studies. Next you will begin data extraction; the first part of this process is deciding what counts as data (Thomas and Harden, 2008). Some would argue for key concepts, some participant quotes; we would recommend considering the results section in its entirety for this first phase. Whatever approach is taken, reviewers should be systematic and consistent in the way they extract data and in their reporting of this. For a more detailed presentation of all possible data extraction methods, please see the relevant chapter on extracting qualitative evidence (Noyes and Lewin, 2011) in *Supplementary Guidance for Inclusion of Qualitative Research in Cochrane Systematic Reviews of Interventions*.

The next step is to analyse and synthesise your evidence. You need to explore the relationships that exist within and across study findings and identify overarching themes and interpretations across studies. As with any other type of synthesis, your analysis is only one interpretation of the data, as it depends on the focus of the review and the perspective of the reviewers; reviewers from different backgrounds may choose to focus on different aspects of the data, or employ different theoretical frameworks to collect, analyse and interpret the findings. Having a multidisciplinary team of reviewers can help increase rigour and develop a richer analysis. In addition, including a reflexive statement, as part of your review paper, where each reviewer explicitly states the assumptions and preconceptions that they bring into the research and that may influence the research process, will allow the reader a better understanding of the synthesis and interpretation of the review findings. An example of this can be found in Kingdon et al. (2018).

There are different methodologies to synthesise qualitative data, such as meta-ethnography (where analysis and synthesis of individual studies should lead to higher order interpretations that were not evident by analysis of the individual studies alone), **grounded theory** synthesis (an inductive approach, often used as a method of theory building) or thematic synthesis. Thematic synthesis (Thomas and Harden, 2008) is one of the most commonly used qualitative synthesis approaches; it is heavily based on the principles of primary qualitative research and shares features with both meta-ethnography and grounded theory.

Thematic synthesis aims to identify recurring ideas or themes in primary studies, to synthesise these descriptively and then to develop these into analytical themes. Initially, using an inductive approach, at least two reviewers independently code, line by line, the qualitative evidence, according to meaning and content. Consequently, these free codes of findings are organised into 'descriptive' themes that encompass the meaning of groups of the initial codes. Finally, based on the codes and 'descriptive' themes and through discussion with the wider review team, the final 'analytical' themes can be developed. These themes can also be presented in a table (together with direct quotations from the primary studies) or as a thematic map, where you visually present your findings and highlight any possible relationships between your themes. See **Table 3.6** for an example of qualitative data used within a thematic synthesis.

Table 3.6 only represents a small part of the thematic synthesis; see the supplementary file for Whitley et al. (2021) for the full thematic synthesis. For a detailed review of the different available methods to synthesise qualitative evidence, see Barnett-Page and Thomas (2009).

Meta-integration

Meta-integration is a technique used to combine the findings from a quantitative *and* a qualitative synthesis. This is needed when performing a systematic mixed studies review. A systematic mixed studies review may synthesise quantitative studies within a meta-analysis, and qualitative studies within a thematic synthesis, and then be left with two separate sets of findings. Meta-integration aims to combine these two sets of findings, perhaps by assessing their complementarity, for example.

Quantitative and qualitative data often address different aspects of a target phenomenon. Therefore, they may not be capable of confirming or refuting each other; instead, their complementarity may be assessed (Sandelowski et al., 2006). Complementarity is found where data are related to each other, linking observations with explanations (Sandelowski et al., 2006) and strengthening the understanding.

Frantzen and Fetters (2016) suggest displaying the meta-integration within a table to illustrate the complex inter-relational connections. This allows identified quantitative variables and qualitative themes to be displayed side by side, along with the conclusion. This not only facilitates the process of meta-integration, but also simplifies the findings for the reader.

Meta-integration Example

We performed a systematic mixed studies review to identify predictors, barriers and facilitators to effective management of acute pain in children by emergency medical services (Whitley et al., 2021). We identified eight quantitative and five qualitative studies and performed a narrative synthesis and thematic synthesis, respectively. We combined the findings of both syntheses within a table and assessed the complementarity. We found that younger children were more likely

Table 3.6 – Thematic synthesis example.

Source quotations	Initial code	Descriptive theme	Analytical theme
'Not only did it relieve some of his pain, but it relieved some of his anxiety. Calmed him down a little bit more. It was easier to deal with him so it does have its benefits' (Williams et al., 2012: 523).	Analgesia improves child anxiety and compliance.	Analgesics are helpful but administration is challenging.	Child factors.
'... We have a lot of barriers to IV access in younger children. The older ones wouldn't be a major problem but certainly younger children, which again certainly affects your mindset in relation to using the likes of morphine ...' (Murphy et al., 2014: 496).	IV access is difficult, especially in younger children.		
'Are you screaming because you're in pain? Are you screaming because you're sad? Are you screaming because you're afraid? Are you screaming because ... well, I don't know' (Gunnvall, et al., 2018: 41).	Assessment of pain is very difficult in children.	Assessment of children is challenging.	
'When you don't know why they are screaming, I think it's hard ...' (Jepsen et al., 2019: 5).			
'How are you going to assess pain in children who cannot communicate, who are too small // Yeah, well, these preverbal children, it's very, very hard to communicate' (Gunnvall et al., 2018: 42).	Younger children are more difficult to assess.		

Source: Whitley et al. (2021).

to achieve effective pain management after the quantitative narrative synthesis. However, we found that younger children were more difficult to assess, cannulate and administer inhaled analgesics to during the thematic synthesis. The overall finding after meta-integration was that the data conflicted each other, and that further research was needed.

Confidence in the Cumulative Evidence

After performing the many steps involved in a systematic review (searching, selecting, extracting, appraising and synthesising), a set of findings and conclusions are generated. It is important to know how much confidence can be placed in these findings. Techniques such as **GRADE** and **GRADE-CERQual** have been developed to assess confidence in the cumulative evidence.

GRADE

The GRADE approach is a system for assessing how much confidence to place in findings from evidence syntheses in quantitative systematic reviews and other evidence syntheses of quantitative data. It is a transparent and systematic way of developing and presenting evidence summaries, as well as developing and assessing the strength of recommendations (including clinical practice guidelines). It should be noted here, though, that systematic reviews are not expected to make such recommendations and, therefore, will not be discussed in length here (GRADE Working Group, 2013).

The GRADE method (Atkins et al., 2004) should be applied to each study outcome across the included studies and it involves six steps:

1. Assigning an a priori ranking of 'high' for randomised controlled trials (RCTs) and 'low' for **observational studies**, based on their likelihood of risk of bias (RCTs are considered less prone to bias)

2. Downgrading or upgrading your initial ranking (based on assessing specific criteria mentioned below)

3. Assigning a final grade for the quality of evidence as 'high', 'moderate', 'low' or 'very low' for each outcome

4. Considering other factors that may have affected the strength of the recommendation, such as cost effectiveness or effect sizes

5. Making final recommendations

6. Overall, the quality of evidence represents a continuum and not discrete categories, and should be interpreted as such.

Reasons for downgrading an initial ranking would be detecting possible methodological and design limitations (that is, risk of bias); inconsistency or heterogeneity of results across studies; indirectness of evidence (such as an indirect comparison of populations, outcomes, interventions, amongst others); imprecision (in both number of events and confidence intervals); and detecting publication bias. On the contrary, reasons for upgrading your initial ranking would be having a large magnitude of effect; when all plausible **confounders** or residual bias increase confidence in the estimated effect (that is, the actual effect is most likely larger than what your evidence is showing); as well as having a dose-response gradient, where the result is proportional to the degree of exposure (that is, having a cause–effect relationship).

For a more detailed description, please see the *GRADE Handbook* (GRADE Working Group, 2013) and Atkins et al. (2004) *Grading quality of evidence and strength of recommendations*.

GRADE-CERQual

The GRADE-CERQual approach (Lewin et al., 2018a) is a system for assessing how much confidence to place in findings from evidence syntheses in qualitative systematic reviews and other evidence syntheses of qualitative data.

Overall, GRADE-CERQual assesses how well your findings represent the phenomenon the review is investigating and involves a transparent assessment of each individual review finding, in terms of four components:

- Methodological limitations
- Coherence
- Adequacy of data
- Relevance.

Methodological limitations refer to any concerns we might have regarding the design and conduct of the studies (that is, the primary studies) that support our review finding. Coherence refers to how accurately and clearly primary studies reflect the phenomenon of interest and how well grounded the finding is in the data from the synthesised primary studies. Adequacy of data refers to whether we have enough data supporting a finding and how rich the data is, whereas relevance refers to whether the data from the synthesised primary studies can be applicable to the context (such as population or setting) of our review question and topic. A fifth area of 'dissemination bias' is currently being considered for addition as well.

Again, as with GRADE, confidence should be assessed for each review finding. Assessments should be described in terms of each of the four components described above and using one of the following levels of concern: 'no or very minor concerns that are unlikely to reduce confidence in the review finding', 'minor concerns that may reduce confidence in the review finding', 'moderate concerns that will probably reduce confidence in the review finding' and 'serious concerns that are very likely to reduce confidence in the review'. Your specific concerns regarding each finding should be described in detail as well. A final grade for the quality of evidence, as 'high', 'moderate', 'low' or 'very low', is assigned as a final step of your assessment. Similar to GRADE for RCTs, all review findings are assigned an a priori ranking of 'high confidence', which might then be rated down, depending on your assessments and whether there are concerns regarding methodological limitations, coherence, adequacy of data and relevance. For a more detailed description, please see Lewin et al. (2018b).

Remember, GRADE and GRADE-CERQual assess the quality of your systematic review findings, not the quality of the individual studies included in your review.

Reporting and Dissemination

There are reporting guidelines for systematic reviews and some journals will require you to submit a checklist (that is, a PRISMA checklist) with your article submission. These checklists can be helpful in shaping your write-up and ensuring that all the correct information is reported.

The abstract for your systematic review should include a brief background with objectives. Your abstract methods should include quite a lot of detail to include data sources, study selection, data extraction, quality assessment and data synthesis. You will likely (dependent on journal guidelines) only have a few sentences for the results and final conclusions, so it is important to get this right. You should not make any speculative statements, and you may wish to include information about the quality of the evidence, as this will affect the confidence in your conclusions/recommendations.

Your introduction should include a concise background, with a summary of evidence to date and a clear rationale and justification for the conduct of your review. The final part of the introduction should be the aim of your systematic review, which will include the key concepts of your review question (such as PICO). The structure and content of your methods and results section will largely be informed by the relevant reporting guidelines/checklists (Moher et al., 2015). The final section, your discussion, should be a fact-based overview of your results, to include the volume and quality of evidence retrieved in addition to a discussion of your main findings. You must only report evidence-based conclusions and recommendations, as it is not appropriate to speculate within this type of discussion (Harris et al., 2013). When writing this section of your review, there should be consideration of the following: the strength of the evidence, theoretical explanations of effectiveness, context as an effect modifier and implications for practice and research (Petticrew and Roberts, 2008).

Having worked hard to conduct your systematic review, it is then important to ensure effective communication of your findings to your target audience (for example, policy makers and practitioners). Often, they may not have time to read the whole review and instead may focus on the abstract and/or the review conclusions. It is important that the conclusions and recommendations are clearly worded and arise directly from the evidence presented in the review. This short piece of text is your opportunity to convey the key findings of your review, the take-home points. When writing your conclusion, ask yourself this question: if the reader were to remember one thing about my review, what should it be?

When planning your dissemination activities, you should think about your target audience and the impact you want your work to have. Your message needs to be clear and accessible, and where possible disseminated via additional platforms beyond that of the academic peer-reviewed journal. Depending on your topic, this may include seminars/workshops, newsletters, direct mailing to policy makers and/or relevant agencies and involvement with local practitioners.

Summary

Conducting a systematic review can be challenging, and the time required and volume of work involved should not be underestimated. The methods must be robust and comprehensive, and they should follow the systematic steps described in this chapter. The reward of producing a high-quality systematic review that may inform clinical practice is worth the effort. If conducting your first systematic review, it is advisable to ensure you have experience on your team by recruiting a researcher who has previously performed a systematic review.

Further Reading

For further guidance on how to develop a review protocol, you can visit the Cochrane Collaboration webpage, where you can access *The Cochrane Handbook for Systematic Reviews of Interventions*: https://training.cochrane.org/handbook

You can also access various published systematic review protocols in *Campbell Systematic Reviews*, an open access journal prepared under the editorial control of the Campbell Collaboration that publishes systematic reviews, methods research papers and evidence and gap maps.

To access a copy of the PRISMA-P checklist, follow this link: http://www.prisma-statement.org/documents/PRISMA-P-checklist.pdf

In addition, you can view a template of a systematic review protocol here: https://endoc.cochrane.org/sites/endoc.cochrane.org/files/public/uploads/CMED_protocol_template.pdf

References

Akobeng, A. K. 2005. Understanding systematic reviews and meta-analysis. *Archives of Disease in Childhood*, 90, 845–848.

Aromataris, E. and Munn, Z. 2020. JBI manual for evidence synthesis. Available at: https://synthesismanual.jbi.global [Accessed 6 October 2020].

Aromataris, E. and Pearson, A. 2014. The systematic review: An overview. *AJN The American Journal of Nursing*, 114, 53–58.

Atkins, D. et al. 2004. Grading quality of evidence and strength of recommendations. *BMJ (Clinical Research Ed.)*, 328, 1490.

Barnett-Page, E. and Thomas, J. 2009. Methods for the synthesis of qualitative research: A critical review. *BMC Medical Research Methodology*, 9, 59.

Bridle, C. 2003. Systematic reviews in health psychology: How and why they should be conducted. *Health Psychology Update*, 12, 3–13.

Buscemi, N. et al. 2006. Single data extraction generated more errors than double data extraction in systematic reviews. *Journal of Clinical Epidemiology*, 59, 697–703.

Campbell, M. et al. 2018. Improving Conduct and reporting Of Narrative Synthesis of Quantitative data (Icons-Quant): Protocol for a mixed methods study to develop a reporting guideline. *BMJ Open*, 8, E020064.

Centre For Reviews and Dissemination. 2008. Systematic reviews. CRD'S guidance for undertaking reviews in health care. Available at: https://www.york.ac.uk/media/crd/systematic_reviews.pdf [Accessed 6 October 2020].

Centre For Reviews and Dissemination. 2020. Prospero. International Prospective Register of Systematic Reviews. University of York. Available at: https://www.crd.york.ac.uk/prospero/ [Accessed 6 October2020].

Curtis, F. et al. 2021. Effects of cognitive behavioural therapy on insomnia in adults with tinnitus: Systematic review and meta-analysis of randomised controlled trials. *Sleep Medicine Reviews*, 56, 101405.

Deeks, J., Higgins, J. and Altman, D. 2020. Chapter 10: Analysing data and undertaking meta-analyses. *In:* Higgins, J. et al. (Eds.) *Cochrane Handbook for Systematic Reviews of Interventions Version 6.1 (Updated September 2020).* Cochrane.

Eaton, G. et al. 2020. Contribution of paramedics in primary and urgent care: A systematic review. *British Journal Of General Practice*, 70, E421–E426.

Engel, G. L. 1977. The need for a new medical model: A challenge for biomedicine. *Science*, 196, 129–136.

Featherstone, R. M. et al. 2015. Advancing knowledge of rapid reviews: An analysis of results, conclusions and recommendations from published review articles examining rapid reviews. *Systematic Reviews*, 4, 50.

Frantzen, K. K. and Fetters, M. D. 2016. Meta-integration for synthesizing data in a systematic mixed studies review: Insights from research on autism spectrum disorder. *Quality and Quantity*, 50, 2251–2277.

Garritty, C. et al. 2020. Cochrane rapid reviews. Interim guidance from the Cochrane Rapid Reviews Methods Group. Available at: https://methods.cochrane.org/rapidreviews/sites/methods .cochrane.org.rapidreviews/files/public/uploads/cochrane_rr_-_guidance-23mar2020-v1.pdf [Accessed 6 October 2020].

Godin, K. et al. 2015. Applying systematic review search methods to the grey literature: A case study examining guidelines for school-based breakfast programs in Canada. *Systematic Reviews*, 4, 138.

Grade Working Group. 2013. GRADE Handbook. Accessed: 10 November 2021. Availble at: https:// gdt.gradepro.org/app/handbook/handbook.html

Gunnvall, K. et al. 2018. Specialist nurses' experiences when caring for preverbal children in pain in the prehospital context in Sweden. *International Emergency Nursing*, 36, 39–45.

Harris, J. D. et al. 2013. How to write a systematic review. *The American Journal of Sports Medicine*, 42, 2761–2768.

Higgins, J. et al. 2002. Statistical heterogeneity in systematic reviews of clinical trials: A critical appraisal of guidelines and practice. *Journal of Health Services Research and Policy*, 7, 51–61.

Jepsen, K., Rooth, K. and Lindstrom, V. 2019. Parents' experiences of the caring encounter in the ambulance service – A qualitative study. *Journal of Clinical Nursing*. 28, 3660–3668.

Jones, A. W. et al. 2017. Systematic review of interventions to improve patient uptake and completion of pulmonary rehabilitation in COPD. *ERJ Open Research*, 3, 00089-2016.

Kingdon, C., Downe, S. and Betran, A. P. 2018. Non-clinical interventions to reduce unnecessary caesarean section targeted at organisations, facilities and systems: Systematic review of qualitative studies. *Plos One*, 13, E0203274.

Lewin, S. et al. 2018a. Applying GRADE-CERQual to qualitative evidence synthesis findings—Paper 2: How to make an overall cerqual assessment of confidence and create a summary of qualitative findings table. *Implementation Science*, 13, 10.

Lewin, S. et al. 2018b. Applying GRADE-CERQual to qualitative evidence synthesis findings: Introduction to the series. *Implementation Science,* 13, 2.

Li, T., Higgins, J. and Deeks, J. 2019. Chapter 5: Collecting data. *In:* Higgins, J., Thomas, J., Chandler, J. et al. (Eds.) *Cochrane Handbook for Systematic Reviews of Interventions Version 6.0 (Updated July 2019).* Cochrane, 2019. Available at: www.training.cochrane.org/handbook.

Moher, D. et al. 2009. Preferred Reporting Items for Systematic reviews and Meta-Analyses: The PRISMA statement. *BMJ*, 339, B2535.

Moher, D. et al. 2015. Preferred Reporting Items for Systematic review and Meta-Analysis Protocols (Prisma-P) 2015 statement. *Systematic Reviews*, 4, 1.

Murphy, A. et al. 2014. A qualitative study of the barriers to prehospital management of acute pain in children. *Emergency Medicine Journal: EMJ*, 31, 493–498.

Noyes, J. and Lewin, S. 2011. Chapter 5: Extracting qualitative evidence. *In:* Noyes, J., Booth, A., Hannes, K. et al. (Eds.) *Supplementary Guidance for Inclusion of Qualitative Research in Cochrane Systematic Reviews of Interventions. Version 1 (Updated August 2011).* Cochrane Collaboration Qualitative Methods Group. Available at: http://cqrmg.cochrane.org/supplemental-handbook-guidance.

Petticrew, M. and Roberts, H. 2008. *Systematic Reviews in the Social Sciences: A Practical Guide.* John Wiley and Sons, New Jersey.

Popay, J. et al. 2006. Guidance on the conduct of narrative synthesis in systematic reviews. A product from the ESRC methods programme. Version 1. Available at: https://www.lancaster.ac.uk/media/lancaster-university/content-assets/documents/fhm/dhr/chir/nssynthesisguidanceversion1-april2006.pdf [Accessed 14 July 2020].

Porritt, K., Gomersall, J. and Lockwood, C. 2014. JBI's systematic reviews: Study selection and critical appraisal. *The American Journal of Nursing*, 114, 47–52.

Ring, N. A. et al. 2011. A Guide to Synthesising Qualitative Research for Researchers Undertaking Health Technology Assessments and Systematic Reviews. Available at: https://dspace.stir.ac.uk/handle/1893/3205.

Sandelowski, M., Voils, C. I. and Barroso, J. 2006. Defining and designing mixed research synthesis studies. *Research in the schools*, 13, 29.

Stewart, L., Moher, D. and Shekelle, P. 2012. Why prospective registration of systematic reviews makes sense. *Systematic Reviews*, 1, 7.

Suarez-Almazor, M. E. et al. 2000. Identifying clinical trials in the medical literature with electronic databases: Medline alone is not enough. *Controlled Clinical Trials*, 21, 476–487.

Thomas, J. and Harden, A. 2008. Methods for the thematic synthesis of qualitative research in systematic reviews. *BMC Medical Research Methodology*, 8, 45.

Tong, A. et al. 2012. ENhancing Transparency in REporting the synthesis of Qualitative research: ENTREQ. *BMC Medical Research Methodology*, 12, 181.

Tricco, A. C. et al. 2018. PRISMA extension for Scoping Reviews (PRISMA-SCR): Checklist AND EXPLANATION. *Annals of Internal Medicine*, 169, 467–473.

Whitley, G. A. et al. 2021. The predictors, barriers and facilitators to effective management of acute pain in children by emergency medical services: A systematic mixed studies review. *Journal of Child Health Care*. 25, 481–503.

Williams, D. M., et al. 2012. Barriers to and enablers for prehospital analgesia for pediatric patients. *Prehospital Emergency Care: Official Journal of the National Association of EMS Physicians and the National Association of State EMS Directors*, 16, 519–526.

Chapter 4

Observational Studies

Tom Quinn

Chapter Objectives

This chapter will cover:

- An overarching definition of observational studies and an introduction to the different study designs that fall within this category
- The position of observational study designs within the hierarchy of evidence
- The strengths and weaknesses of observational studies compared with other methods
- Published standards for reporting observational studies
- Examples of observational studies from the urgent and emergency care literature

---

Introduction

Observational studies have several roles in improving the evidence base for clinical practice and service delivery. These include addressing research questions that are not suitable for **randomised controlled trials**, monitoring for longer term effects of interventions that occur beyond the follow-up period in randomised trials and providing preliminary data to inform trials. Observational methods also provide important epidemiological evidence, for example, in identifying associations of **outcomes** with risk factor exposures. In clinical practice, observational studies provide information about associations between an exposure (such as a new intervention or pathway) and an outcome of interest (such as mortality, admission to hospital), but are not generally able to infer causation.

This chapter will provide an overview of observational methods; discuss the strengths and limitations compared to randomised trials, including conventions and language used to describe and report study findings, particularly in relation to attribution of causation; and provide examples from the literature.

What Is an Observational Study?

The hallmark of observational methods is that patients (or their data) are observed, without the investigator altering treatments or pathways of care. Thus, observational studies do not entail experiments.

Importantly, in contrast to randomised trials, observational studies have the potential to provide 'real-world' evidence beyond the restrictions of trial inclusion and exclusion criteria and may therefore provide more generalisable estimates of the effects of a particular intervention. A recent example of how observational studies can complement completed randomised controlled trials was shown in the SARS-CoV-2 pandemic, when large observational studies provided reassurance about the effectiveness of various vaccines in 'real-world' practice that had been shown to be efficacious in the more restricted trial population (Dagan et al., 2021).

Observational studies dominate the evidence base in many aspects of modern medicine. For example, the American Heart Association 2020 guidelines for cardiopulmonary resuscitation contain 491 recommendations, of which 20% are based on non-randomised studies, 51% are based on limited data (such as small, single-centre studies, case reports or animal studies) and 17% on expert opinion. A mere 1% are based on multiple randomised trials or **systematic reviews** of trials, and 15% on a single trial (Merchant et al., 2020). The picture is only slightly better across over 50 authoritative guidelines comprising over 6,000 recommendations published by the American College of Cardiology (ACC), American Heart Association (AHA) and European Society of Cardiology (ESC) (Fanaroff et al., 2019). Only a small percentage were supported by evidence from multiple randomised controlled trials (RCTs) or a single, large RCT, a pattern that did not meaningfully improve from 2008 to 2018. A review of articles published in emergency medicine journals over a 20-year period reported no change in the proportion of experimental studies (such as randomised trials) between 1997 and 2017 (Smith et al., 2020). Thus, observational studies continue to dominate the emergency medicine literature.

Types of Observational Study

The main types of observational study designs are **cohort studies, cross-sectional studies** and **case-control studies**. In recent years, powerful new opportunities to conduct observational research using routinely collected data in administrative datasets and disease-specific registries have gained popularity.

Form follows function. The chosen research methods depend upon the research question that is being addressed. For example, a research team seeking to address a question about the prevalence of, say, 999 calls involving people with seizures might choose to use a cross-sectional study, whereas if the question relates to the incidence of a condition then a cohort design would be appropriate. **Box 4.1** sets out the common objectives and some indicative examples of study design.

Box 4.1: Common Objectives and Study Design

Objective	Example of study design
To estimate treatment effects	Randomised controlled trial
To estimate prevalence	Cross-sectional study
To estimate incidence	Cohort study
To estimate association of exposure with outcome	Cohort study

Definition and Different Types of Observational Study Design

Hierarchy of Evidence

Observational studies are ranked below randomised trials in the '**hierarchy of evidence**' (see **Chapter 1: Introduction, Figure 1.1**). When RCTs are performed using standard design characteristics, the intervention under study is the only variable that differs between the groups. As such, RCTs are much better suited to establishing causality in the specific population studied than observational studies. Because study outcomes, predictors and **confounding** variables can be better measured and controlled in prospective cohort studies, they are ranked higher than retrospective studies. Case-control studies are ranked below cohort studies. In respect to observational studies of interventions, these are frequently considered to generate new hypotheses that are likely to require confirmation by randomised trial (Bowman et al., 2020).

Cohort Studies

In cohort studies, a group of participants with an exposure of interest and a group without the exposure are identified. Both groups are followed up over time to observe outcomes. When this is undertaken prospectively, the assumption is that the exposure preceded the outcome. This method is useful in facilitating calculations such as incidence rates and relative risks, amongst others, but when event rates are very low or even rare, longer follow-up – even over several years – may be necessary, with all that implies for the cost and complexity of undertaking the research. The risk of loss to follow-up of study participants is an acknowledged limitation.

Another form of cohort study is undertaken retrospectively, using participants with an outcome of interest and looking backwards over time, for example using **chart review** methods, discussed in more detail below. This method is commonly employed in emergency care research. By their nature, such studies tend to be cheaper and more efficient, because the data have already been collected before the study starts, and are (subject to institutional and sometimes ethics committee approvals) readily available. However, these perceived advantages need to be balanced with the disadvantages of the study data having been collected for purposes other than the specific research question being addressed, with attendant risks that the dataset may be incomplete or important variables may not have been collected as part of the routine patient record, or simply be missing.

Put simply, prospective cohort studies 'look ahead' to study outcomes, while retrospective studies 'look back' from the outcomes (Schulz and Grimes, 2019).

In cohort studies, inability to control for all the factors that might differ between study participants is an important source of **bias**. This means that so-called 'confounding variables' may not be taken into account during analysis because they are unknown or missing, or simply not measured (eloquently termed 'lurking factors' by Spiegelhalter (2019)). It is therefore important to carefully consider the approach to analysis of the data (preferably with the advice of a statistician, working with clinical and methodological experts) before commencing the study.

Chart Review

Put simply, chart reviews are studies in which information is abstracted from the medical records, whether paper or electronic. In chart reviews, the data have already been collected as part of routine clinical documentation, thus they are analogous to retrospective cohort studies. Chart review studies are common in emergency medicine research, being the method of choice in over half of original studies published in emergency medical service journals and a quarter of articles in emergency medicine speciality journals (Kaji et al., 2014). While this method brings advantages of convenience and speed, and reduces the costs associated with prospective data collection, there are several disadvantages. Not least being the quality of documentation during routine clinical care, an issue which is a known phenomenon in prehospital care, for example, in the quality of clinicians' documentation of reasons for non-conveyance (Porter et al., 2008), patient physiology following motor vehicle accidents (Laudermilch et al., 2010; Staff and Søvik, 2011) and recognition of sepsis (Latten et al., 2020). Whether the introduction of electronic patient records in prehospital care will result in more complete documentation remains an area for further investigation (Porter et al., 2020).

Documentation serves several purposes, for example, being a record of the assessment and care of individual patients; providing sources for monitoring activity for administrative, costing and contracting purposes; and informing investigations in the event of serious incidents or complaints. Routine health records are rarely designed with research (and certainly not a specific research question) in mind. Thus, key variables may be missing because of poor documentation practices as described above, or simply because the variables of interest for a particular research project are not present on the patient record in the first place.

The processes for chart review have been described by Kaji et al. (2014). These are intended to address ten potential sources (or 'layers') of bias to improve the quality of chart review studies. The principles espoused by Kaji et al. (2014) are used below (although some of the headings have been modified for this chapter) to consider in more detail key requirements for ensuring quality when designing and conducting observational research in prehospital care.

Are the Available Data and Chosen Research Design Appropriate to Address the Research Question?

Any data to be collected and analysed need to be representative of the patient population being studied. Thus, for prehospital studies, the comprehensiveness and quality of documentation in routine ambulance records is a key consideration. For example, will there be sufficient patients with the condition of interest to make the study feasible and worthwhile? An example might be a rare disease such as Vascular type Ehlers-Danlos syndrome (Busch et al., 2016), which an individual clinician or service is unlikely to encounter with sufficient frequency to provide the data on which to draw any inferences about presenting characteristics, treatment or outcomes: thus, collaborative studies drawing data from across multiple organisations and systems would be required.

Another key consideration is the availability of the required variables to inform any statistical modelling. For example, studying the History, ECG, Age, Risk Factors and Troponin (HEART) score (Six et al., 2013), designed for use in the emergency department for prediction of major adverse cardiac events, would be unlikely to be informative in patients presenting in the prehospital setting with chest pain given that troponin tests are not currently available in most emergency medical service settings. Where point of care troponin testing is available, however, undertaking such a study has been possible (Stopyra et al., 2020).

A mere 10% of published chart review studies in emergency medicine reported a sample size calculation (Badcock et al., 2005).

Study-specific documentation, including data collection/abstraction forms, should be developed, piloted and shared as part of subsequent dissemination of study findings, for example, as an online appendix to a published paper. This is increasingly required by journal editors.

Investigator Bias and Transparency

One of the fundamental tenets of research integrity is transparency. Researchers should declare any conflicts (or potential conflicts) of interest, whether financial or philosophical. An example of the former might be receiving honoraria from a commercial entity such as a device manufacturer. An example of the latter is where the researcher already believes strongly in the exposure under study, be that a device, medicine or new pathway, or is seeking to 'prove' the values of something they are emotionally invested in. Such declarations should be made when applying for organisational, ethical or other approvals, and when disseminating study findings.

Representativeness of the Study Population

Researchers should establish clear inclusion and exclusion criteria before data collection commences. A flow diagram should be provided to show how the study population (participants, sample) was derived from the source population, for example, using the study flow diagrams presented in the **STROBE** or **RECORD** reporting methods (discussed later in this chapter).

Internal and External Validity

Internal validity refers to the strength of the inferences from the study: is the exposure or intervention associated with a difference in the outcome (high internal validity) or was there a systematic error in the study that influenced any difference in the outcome (low internal validity)? Can any observed changes found in the study be attributed to the exposure and not to other possible causes? The absence of a control group or having a control group that is not comparable to the exposure (or intervention) group – different baseline characteristics, for example, or even unmeasured differences – may compromise the internal validity of a study. Internal validity in and of itself is a prerequisite for **external validity**.

Small, single-centre observational studies, common in the prehospital literature, are frequently noted to have low external validity. External validity refers to the ability to generalise study findings to a wider population: the degree to which study conclusions might apply to people in other places and at other times.

Variables to Be Collected

Careful attention to data collection is important to reduce potential bias through multiple conflicting entries, interpretations, miscoding or misclassification. Study variables should be clearly defined and documented and coding rules confirmed before data collection begins. Research staff abstracting data from patient records should receive training in study-specific definitions and procedure. An example of this can be found in Gavalova et al. (2019), where research paramedics in three ambulance services were trained in data abstraction processes specific to a study of the prehospital 12-lead electrocardiogram. Details of such processes should be provided as an appendix to any study outputs.

Systematic Data Collection

As discussed above, it is useful to have a standardised study proforma that sets out uniformly the variables that are to be abstracted from any case notes, including specific data definitions to avoid misclassification. This should be piloted prior to formal data collection commencing. The data collection instrument should, where possible, be electronic to reduce the risk of data entry errors. An example of a commercially available instrument is the Research Electronic Data Capture system (REDCap) developed by Vanderbilt University (Patridge and Bardyn, 2018).

Missing Data

Missing data are a common feature of observational studies and can threaten study validity. Measures should be established during the study design phase to address missing data, including careful development (with the involvement or advice of a statistician) of the study statistical analysis plan (SAP), setting out clearly how missing data will be assessed (to determine to what extent it is missing, whether this is at random or not) and how this will be dealt with through techniques such as multiple imputation. Lee et al. (2021) propose a framework for Treatment And Reporting of Missing data in Observational Studies (TARMOS).

Abstractor Bias

Research staff responsible for data collection or abstraction are not immune to bias and should ideally be blinded to study objectives and hypotheses, although in practice this principle has rarely been adhered to (Kaji et al., 2014; Worster et al., 2005). Abstractor bias is particularly likely when the study team is small and unfunded and the researchers are themselves responsible for data abstraction.

Training and Supporting Research Staff Abstracting Data

Whoever is responsible for collecting or abstracting data, training will be required to ensure consistency of approach and to maintain study quality. In many studies, data are abstracted by health professionals (research paramedics for example), but it is not unusual for this responsibility to rest with research staff with no clinical training, who may be less familiar with the source documentation (such as how the ambulance report form is set out), which increases the risk of misinterpretation of clinical terms or jargon, misinterpretation of test results or other factors that may result in erroneous data entry. Electronic patient records may mitigate these challenges, but abstractor familiarity with the system being used is essential. Given these considerations, abstractors should receive standardised training in study procedures (if needs be, for longer term studies, with periodic refresher training) to ensure uniformity of approach, and have contact details for study co-ordinators or the principal investigator to ensure rapid resolution of queries. Regular team meetings to discuss study progress, to resolve or clarify coding issues and for quality monitoring are recommended.

Assessing Abstractor Reliability

Abstractor (or rater) reliability is an important consideration in observational research as it represents the extent to which the data collected are correct representations of the variables measured. Where multiple team members are abstracting data for a study, then measurement of the extent to which they consistently assign the same scores (or codes) to the same variables is termed **inter-rater reliability**. While training in study procedures, a study manual outlining agreed procedures, definitions and coding practices can help with consistent approaches by abstractors. It is accepted practice that the level of agreement is quantified using a statistic such as Cohen's kappa (Kaji et al., 2014). Where a single person is abstracting data, the consistency of their approach is important (are they consistently recording/coding the same variables in the same way, for example). A detailed discussion of these issues is beyond the scope of this chapter but there are several helpful texts, such as McHugh (2012), which are informative. As always, expert advice from a statistician should be sought.

Reflective Questions

When designing an observational study, have you considered the appropriateness of the choice of design to addressing your research question?

How might you prepare research assistants, paramedics or other study staff to abstract data if using chart review methods? What measures do you need to put in place to ensure consistency and quality of data collection?

On completing your observational study, and preparing for publication of findings, what key terms should be avoided to ensure that a causal relationship between exposure and outcome is not suggested?

Case-control Studies

In the case-control study, people with and without a condition of interest are identified and data from their clinical records (and possibly other sources such as asking them to complete questionnaires on lifestyle or other areas of interest) are analysed.

Since case-control studies are by their nature retrospective, they can be relatively inexpensive and can be conducted rapidly. Loss to follow-up is therefore not something that is encountered. It is also possible to examine several exposures in relation to a single condition. The case-control design is useful in studying rare disorders or events, largely because undertaking a prospective cohort study requiring an unrealistically large sample size and follow-up for a prolonged period would be expensive and probably unfeasible.

However, case-control studies are unsuitable for researching exposures that are uncommon. They have the potential to suffer from recall and **selection bias** (selection of cases and controls requires particular attention to ensure that participants from both groups come from the target population of interest), and they include a specified number of cases and controls so it is not possible to obtain either prevalence or incidence. In interpreting the findings of case-control studies, it can sometimes be challenging to determine causality, that is, whether the exposure occurred prior to the outcome of interest.

Two sources of data are required – one for the cases (patients with the condition of interest) and one for controls (patients without the condition of interest). Cases can be identified from a variety of sources such as clinical records or administrative databases, registries (discussed in more detail later in this chapter), death certificates or population surveys.

Whether the condition of interest for a particular study has been newly diagnosed or the patient has had the condition for some time prior to the study starting is an important consideration when considering assessment of causality. Someone with existing or longstanding disease may have had multiple relevant exposures since their initial diagnosis; therefore, careful consideration must be given to this in study design and conduct.

Sources of controls vary, depending on resource and time availability. Examples include patient records held by ambulance services, primary care, hospitals or disease-specific registries. Where the source has very large numbers of patient records, it might be appropriate given resource constraints to randomly select a sample on the basis of practicality.

While randomised controlled trials can achieve a balance across patient characteristics in each study arm, this is more difficult in observational studies. Adjustments for differences in potential confounding factors will therefore be necessary as part of the statistical analysis. Cases and controls are selected on the basis of their status with respect to the condition of interest, and the intention of the study is to compare the two groups in terms of exposures of interest. Therefore, those with (cases) and without (controls) would be expected to have different characteristics, but controls should be similar to cases in all important respects except of course for not having the outcome of interest. Attempts should be made when the study is designed to prespecify factors known to be **confounders**, such as age, sex and smoking status (a process known as matching).

It is important that data to be collected are specified clearly ('prespecified') as part of the study design process. Standard definitions and diagnostic criteria should be used. The same methods for identifying and measuring exposures should be used to avoid bias. Assessment of exposures should be undertaken by researchers blinded to the status of the study participant (whether they are in the case or control group), especially where the researcher is collecting data direct from study participants (or their proxies, such as a family member, where the patient lacks capacity or has died), for example, by conducting interviews or completing questionnaires. The potential for recall bias in case-control studies must be taken into consideration when seeking information from study participants. People with the condition are often better at remembering past details (such as exposures) than people without the condition; it is also possible of course that someone who has been very ill (such as cardiac arrest or sustained traumatic brain injury) may have difficulty in accurately remembering key exposures or details preceding the event.

A search while preparing this chapter revealed few examples of published case-control studies in the prehospital literature. Charlton et al. (2020) reported a case-control study to determine the effectiveness of intravenous versus oral paracetamol in the management of acute pain in the out-of-hospital setting. Data on 40 patients over 18 years of age transported by ambulance to the Emergency Department (ED), and who received 1 gram of intravenous paracetamol, were extracted from ambulance electronic records, and case matched by sex and age with 40 consecutive patients who received 1 gram of oral paracetamol over the same time period. The primary outcome was the mean reduction in pain score using the numeric rating scale (NRS), with a reduction of 2 or more accepted as clinically significant. Patients receiving intravenous paracetamol had a clinically significant mean improved pain score compared to those receiving oral paracetamol, and 13/40 (32.5%) patients who received intravenous paracetamol saw an improved pain score of $\geq$ 2 compared to 8/40 (20%) who received oral paracetamol. The authors suggested that further evaluation using 'more robust' methods would be necessary to confirm their findings. One example that may be of interest to the prehospital reader is that of O'Neill et al. (2019), who examined the relationships between ED attendances, hospital admissions and death by suicide over a five-year period in Northern Ireland, using patient records from hospital administrative data. Each person who died by suicide (cases) was matched to five living patients (controls), based on age and sex. Death by suicide was associated with recent ED attendance, recent hospital admission and living in a more deprived or urban area, suggesting that ED staff have an important role to play in suicide prevention.

An example of a case-control study from the wider literature is that of a large food poisoning outbreak in nursery and primary schools in Southern Italy during 2018. The researchers used questionnaires to collect information on dates of symptom onset, type and duration of symptoms, healthcare contact, school attendance and food consumed during school lunch breaks. Through information gained on pupils who did (cases) and did not (controls) have food poisoning, a particular batch of cheese from two suppliers was identified as the most likely exposure, and genomic analysis was able to confirm that the cheese was the vehicle of infection (Sorgentone et al., 2021).

Cross-sectional Studies

A cross-sectional study is an observational study that looks at data from a population at one specific point in time, providing a 'snapshot' to allow estimation of prevalence of a given condition, service or other outcome, meaning the proportion of individuals in a population who have a particular disease or service need at a given time. Both exposure and outcome are studied simultaneously. A well-known use of cross-sectional study design is the Household Census, which is sent to every household in the UK; answers to the census questions help government organisations make decisions on planning and funding public services, including transport, education and healthcare. Cross-sectional studies are common in the prehospital literature.

In healthcare, this study design is frequently used to support the planning of services for particular patient groups. For example, Dickson et al. (2016) undertook a cross-sectional study using routinely collected data from the Yorkshire Ambulance Service over a 12-month period, and a consecutive series of individual incidents from the city of Sheffield during the month of May 2012, to document the clinical characteristics of patients with suspected seizures. They described the patients' prehospital management and immediate outcomes and estimated the cost of emergency care, to inform a programme of research to develop new models of care. The authors reported that the majority of patients with suspected seizures encountered by the ambulance service during the study period were transported to hospital, suggesting improvements could be made to the patient pathway. McLachlan et al. (2021) surveyed critical care paramedics over a period of 52 nights to ascertain demand for prehospital critical care services during night hours in two counties served by a single air ambulance, identifying an unmet need for out-of-hours critical care provision. Siriwardena et al. (2019) used a cross-sectional design to identify how patient and paramedic characteristics affected the treatment of pain in two regional ambulance services in England. Records for all eligible adult patients transported to hospital following an ambulance call during one week in April 2016 were analysed. While no association was found between patient sex, or the sex or grade of ambulance staff and use of analgesia or pain reduction, the authors reported that initial pain scores were missing in 42% of patients, even where analgesia was documented as having been administered, suggesting the need for further research and improvement activity in relation to prehospital pain management.

Voss et al. (2018) conducted a retrospective cross-sectional study of patient records from two UK ambulance services of calls to patients aged 65 years and over during 24- or 48-hour periods in January 2017 and July 2017. Two researchers used a standard template to extract data from 3,037 records using a coding structure. Dementia was recorded in 421 records (13.9%). Patients with dementia were significantly less likely to be conveyed to hospital than those without dementia, but call-cycle times were similar for patients regardless of whether or not they had dementia. Calls to people with dementia were more likely to be due to injury following a fall, with the authors concluding that hospital conveyance rates for older people may be related to comorbidities, frailty and complex needs, rather than dementia.

An example of where a cross-sectional design can be employed to rapidly obtain valuable information across multiple countries, without a significant resource requirement to conduct the study, is that of the Euro Heart Survey. Member countries of the European Society of Cardiology (ESC) were invited to participate in a one-week survey of all patients admitted for acute myocardial infarction (AMI). Data on baseline characteristics, type of AMI, management and complications were recorded using a dedicated electronic form, together with data collected during the same time period in national registries in Sweden, England and Wales. Overall, in 4,236 patients from 47 participating countries, of which 60% of patients in the study had documented ST-segment elevation MI, in-hospital mortality was 6.2%. Regional differences were observed in terms of population characteristics, management and outcomes, but these were judged to have moderate influence on patient outcomes (Puymirat et al., 2013).

The main advantage of cross-sectional studies is that they can be conducted relatively quickly and cheaply compared to other study designs. They do however have several disadvantages, including the inability to estimate incidence of a condition, risk of low response rates and recall bias if surveys or interviews are used. In the McLachlan et al. (2021) study, for example, only 11 of 17 critical care paramedics invited to participate did so. There may also have been differences in the characteristics of the non-responding paramedics, such as the geographical area they worked in and types of incidents attended, and the inability to establish a temporal relationship between exposure and outcome.

Bias and Confounding

Bias has a specific meaning in the context of research. While the common usage of the term is taken to denote some form of prejudice, bias undermines the internal validity of research through systematic (as opposed to random) deviation from the scientific truth. The lack of internal validity, or incorrect assessment of the estimated association between an exposure and an effect in the target population, does not therefore represent the true value. Some lists of potential biases comprise as many as 74 categories (Delgado-Rodríguez and Llorca, 2004); the commonest are summarised in **Box 4.2**.

Confounding

Confounding is an inaccuracy or distortion in the estimated measure of association that occurs when the primary exposure of interest is mixed up with some other (extraneous) factor or factors that are associated with the outcome, such that participants in one group differ fundamentally from another group in relation to the likelihood of experiencing the outcome of interest in a study. Confounding by indication arises when a study participant receiving a treatment or intervention is inherently different from someone who is not receiving the treatment or intervention, because there must be a reason the former is having the treatment. For example, Sakurai et al. (2019) compared the data of patients with out-of-hospital cardiac arrest (OCHA) with confirmed cardiac output on Emergency Medical Services (EMS) arrival and considered the confounding factors in prehospital airway management studies. The proportion of patients with confirmed cardiac output on EMS arrival was significantly higher in the bag valve mask (BVM) group than in the advanced airway management (AAM) group. The proportion of patients with favourable neurological outcomes was 30% (117/386) in those with cardiac output on EMS arrival compared with 1.8% (223/12481) in those without.

When confirmed cardiac output on EMS arrival was added to the multivariable model analysis, the OR for a good neurological outcome with BVM decreased from 3.24 (2.49 to 4.20) to 2.60 (1.97 to 3.44) (Sakurai et al., 2019).

In randomised trials, known and unknown confounders may be expected to be evenly balanced across intervention and comparator groups, because of the **randomisation** process. In observational studies, where there is, by definition, no random allocation, the lack of comparability between groups may bias estimates

Box 4.2: Types of Bias in Observational Research

Selection bias: study participants are not representative of the population of interest.

Responder bias: study participants may have different characteristics to those who choose not to participate (or decline consent for their data to be used).

Recall bias: study participants may be more (or less) likely to accurately remember information about past events or exposures.

Withdrawal bias: participants who elect to leave a study (for example, they no longer wish to complete follow-up assessments) may differ from those who do not, risking distortion of the results.

Assessment bias: using different definitions of outcomes or means of collecting and recording them by researchers according to different participant characteristics.

Measurement bias: differences in measuring or recording study exposures according to participant outcomes.

Observer bias: how (and which) questions might be asked by researchers if they are aware of the participant's health status compared to if they are 'blinded' to the information.

Immortal time bias: when an exposure is defined after a participant enters a study, they will be 'immortal' until the exposure occurs. If the participant dies after study **enrolment** but before receiving the exposure (such as a treatment or intervention), they will be classed as unexposed.

A type of bias of particular interest to prehospital researchers is resuscitation time bias. Since interventions (for example, tracheal intubation or administration of intravenous adrenaline) are more likely to be required the longer the duration of a resuscitation attempt, the length of time of the cardiac arrest is causally related to the intervention. Since a longer duration of cardiac arrest is associated with worse patient outcomes, the effect of intra-arrest interventions will be biased towards a harmful effect (Andersen et al., 2018).

of associations between exposure and outcome; statistical techniques are required to account for this. These include matching, multivariable regression, stratification, instrumental variables and propensity score analysis. Detailed statistical techniques are beyond the scope of this chapter, but the key elements are summarised in **Table 4.1**. Statistical methods for observational studies are discussed in more detail by other authors (Andersen and Kurth, 2018; Morshed et al., 2009). The importance of seeking expert advice from a statistician when planning a study is emphasised.

Table 4.1 – Statistical techniques to address confounding in observational studies.

Method	Key points	Advantages	Disadvantages
Matching	Confounders are identified and participants in the groups are matched on the basis of these. Thus, the two groups are 'the same' in relation to these factors.	Simple and efficient.	Reduces available sample size and study power (especially if matched variables are not true confounders). Risk of 'over matching'. Cannot explore associations with matched variables.
Multivariable adjustment/ regression	Mathematical relationships between two or more variables are modelled. Allows estimation of association between dependent and independent variables, while controlling for influence of other independent variables. • For binary outcomes (such as prevalence), a logistic regression model is used and the effect estimated is expressed as an odds ratio (OR). • For continuous outcomes (such as a functional outcome score following cardiac arrest), a linear regression model is used and the estimate of effect is expressed as mean difference. • For time-to-event outcomes (such as 'call-to-needle' in stroke patients), Cox proportional hazards are used and estimate of effect is expressed as a hazard ratio (HR). • Where rate is the outcome (such as rates of ambulance utilisation), Poisson regression is used and the estimate of effect is expressed as the rate ratio.	Allows efficient, simultaneous adjustment for multiple confounders.	The quality of estimates will be reliant on assumptions and fit of the chosen model.

Stratification	Confounding (or potential confounding) variables are identified and the study cohort is grouped by levels of this factor; further analyses are performed on those subgroups of the cohort within which the factor remains constant.	Simple to apply. Modification of effects easy to identify.	While useful when only one or two confounders, it is more difficult to manage and interpret when there are multiple confounders.
Instrumental variable	If a variable can be identified that may cause variation in exposure of interest but has no impact on outcome, it is possible to estimate the magnitude of such variation and its effect on outcome.	Unconfounded estimates can be produced without the need to identify all possible confounders.	Inferences can only be drawn from participants whose exposure is impacted by the instrumental variable.
Propensity score analysis	Two stage process: the probability of exposure (to receiving the intervention) is modelled, with possible confounding variables taken into account. This probability is the propensity score, ranging from 0 to 1. This score is then generated for each participant and used to 'match' them or perform stratified analysis. Can be used in multivariable regression along with exposure variable to estimate outcome.	More robust to modelling assumptions. May be useful where outcomes are rare.	Risk of bias from unknown and unmeasured confounders. Advantages over multivariable adjustment/regression have been questioned.

Registries and Observational Research

Disease-specific registries, often 'owned' and developed by specialist medical societies, have several roles, including the assessment of the translation of findings from randomised trials into routine clinical care of patients. They also track adoption of evidence-based strategies and implementation of guidelines, in some cases identifying low adoption rates or, on a more positive note, providing evidence of improvement (Cohen et al., 2015; McNamara, 2010).

As has already been discussed, the use of routine clinical or administrative datasets has its limitations, including that not every variable of interest will have been collected in relation to a specific research question. An example of this is Quinn et al. (2014), who undertook a secondary analysis of the Myocardial Ischaemia National Audit Project (MINAP) database covering England and Wales, to explore the use of the prehospital 12-lead electrocardiogram (PHECG) in patients hospitalised with acute coronary syndrome. While this study was able to quantify the proportion of patients seen by ambulance clinicians who subsequently underwent PHECG and to estimate associations between the procedure and both patient outcomes and processes of care, it was unable to explore factors such as patient presentation (for example, nature of pain and other symptoms), the influence of patients' and/or ambulance clinicians' sex and other potential confounders as these were not recorded in the MINAP dataset. Moreover, responsibility for inputting data to MINAP rested with hospitals rather than with the ambulance services who cared for the patients, with the risk that the use of PHECG was underestimated compared to actual practice. Such issues are therefore being addressed through a mixed methods study (Gavalova et al., 2019), which includes two further work packages, extending the research beyond the original quantitative secondary analysis undertaken in the original study. One of these work packages is a qualitative study of the influences on EMS clinicians associated with recording PHECG or not. The other comprises a retrospective chart review of ambulance records.

Registries also have a role in providing information on how treatments are provided to patients who have been excluded from trials or who are not represented in adequate numbers in them. As discussed previously, clinical trial participants, or indeed participating research sites, are not always representative of patients with the condition of interest, or the organisations caring for them, whether this be in their baseline characteristics or in outcomes. An example of this would be in relation to provision of primary percutaneous coronary intervention (PPCI) for patients with acute ST-elevation myocardial infarction treated in tertiary centres with a strong research culture, and non-specialist centres who may have less research infrastructure and experience of recruiting patients to complex trials, and of course the experience of conditions in relation to the condition of interest and any intervention.

Specialist, disease-specific registries in the UK and abroad have provided useful insights through observational studies, for example, in determining patient and health service factors associated with variations in hospital mortality following resuscitation from out-of-hospital cardiac arrest (Couper et al., 2018), and recently, from Sweden, characteristics and outcomes of in- and out-of-hospital cardiac arrest in patients with and without COVID-19 during the first wave of the pandemic (Sultanian et al., 2021).

As with other observational study designs, disease registries have limitations in relation to internal validity. For example, if participating centres or clinicians have different thresholds for providing an intervention or treatment (such as taking a patient to the cardiac catheter laboratory or admitting them to the intensive care unit), there is the risk of confounding by indication. An example of where this might be important is in relation to the baseline risk of patients, with those at high risk of an adverse outcome sometimes not being offered the relevant intervention, with all this implies for comparing outcomes.

External validity can similarly be affected by selection bias in registries. We know, for example, that not all patients with a diagnosis of myocardial infarction are included in MINAP (Herrett et al., 2013).

Observational studies may be useful for assessing whether an RCT is feasible. For example, electronic databases or registries can be interrogated to estimate the number of patients who might meet trial eligibility criteria. They may also provide an efficient means of identifying and facilitating recruitment of patients to RCTs, and of facilitating follow-up of outcomes against pre-defined clinical endpoints. Such approaches have the potential to reduce the cost and complexity of RCTs, but there are caveats. The potential lack of quality, accuracy and completeness of observational datasets whose primary purpose was not that of a specific RCT is an important shortcoming. But there are examples of where the 'registry-based randomised trial' has been successful and significantly less costly than the traditional RCT in cardiology; for example, Hofmann et al. (2017) used the Swedish Web system for Enhancement and Development of Evidence-based care in Heart disease Evaluated According to Recommended Therapies (SWEDEHEART) registry as the platform to conduct a large RCT assessing the effects of supplementary oxygen therapy in patients with suspected acute myocardial infarction. In the UK, the PARAMEDIC trial investigators assessed the **feasibility** of using national administrative and clinical datasets (Hospital Episode Statistics (HES), the Intensive Care National Audit and Research Centre, the Myocardial Ischaemia National Audit Project and the National Audit of Percutaneous Coronary Interventions) to follow up patients transported to hospital following attempted resuscitation in a cluster randomised trial of a mechanical chest compression device in out-of-hospital cardiac arrest. They reported that it is feasible to track patients from the prehospital setting through to hospital admission using routinely available administrative datasets with a moderate to high degree of success (Ji et al., 2018).

> ## Box 4.3 Examples of Appropriate Terms Based on Study Design
>
> For randomised controlled trials:
>
> 'The [intervention] reduced the risk of [outcome]'.
>
> 'The [intervention] was more effective than [control/comparator]'.
>
> 'The [intervention] caused [outcome]'.
>
> For observational studies:
>
> 'A lower risk of [outcome] was observed'.
>
> 'There was an association between [exposure] and [outcome]'.

Reporting Outcomes From Observational Studies: Language Matters

The language used in reporting outcomes from observational studies has received attention in recent years. Given the inherent limitations of observational studies, despite the use of statistical techniques such as multivariate adjustment and propensity score analysis, it is not possible for researchers to adjust for many baseline differences (and of course unknown or unrecognised confounders will not be considered). It is therefore considered inappropriate in an observational study to attribute a causal effect of an intervention to an outcome (Kohli and Cannon, 2012). Examples of the types of language to consider when reporting different study types are shown in **Box 4.3**.

Reporting Guidelines for Observational Studies

The Enhancing the QUAlity and Transparency Of health Research (**EQUATOR**) network is an international initiative seeking to improve the reliability and value of published health research by promoting transparent and accurate reporting. Reporting guidelines provide a structured approach to help researchers writing manuscripts for publication and assist those reading published research as well as those seeking to replicate a study. Standardised reporting of research studies also helps those incorporating studies into a systematic review. Lack of adherence to reporting guidelines can result in retraction of published studies, as described by Benchimol et al. (2020) in the context of the rush to publish during the COVID-19 pandemic.

For observational studies, the pertinent reporting guidelines are STROBE (Strengthening The Reporting of OBservational studies in Epidemiology) (von Elm et al., 2014) and RECORD, the latter standing for the REporting of studies Conducted using Observational Routinely collected health Data (Benchimol et al., 2015). Details of the key elements of the STROBE and RECORD reporting criteria are shown in **Box 4.4**.

Box 4.4 STROBE and RECORD Reporting Criteria

STROBE Reporting Criteria

	Item no.	Recommendation	Page no.
Title and abstract	1	(a) Indicate the study's design with a commonly used term in the title or the abstract.	
		(b) Provide in the abstract an informative and balanced summary of what was done and what was found.	
Introduction			
Background/ rationale	2	Explain the scientific background and rationale for the investigation being reported.	
Objectives	3	State specific objectives, including any prespecified hypotheses.	
Methods			
Study design	4	Present key elements of study design early in the paper.	
Setting	5	Describe the setting, locations and relevant dates, including periods of recruitment, exposure, follow-up and data collection.	
Participants	6	(a) *Cohort study* – Give the eligibility criteria, and the sources and methods of selection of participants. Describe methods of follow-up. *Case-control study* – Give the eligibility criteria, and the sources and methods of case ascertainment and control selection. Give the rationale for the choice of cases and controls. *Cross-sectional study* – Give the eligibility criteria, and the sources and methods of selection of participants.	
		(b) *Cohort study* – For matched studies, give matching criteria and number of exposed and unexposed. *Case-control study* – For matched studies, give matching criteria and the number of controls per case.	

(continued)

Box 4.4 STROBE and RECORD Reporting Criteria (*continued*)

	Item no.	Recommendation	Page no.
Variables	7	Clearly define all outcomes, exposures, predictors, potential confounders and effect modifiers. Give diagnostic criteria, if applicable.	
Data sources/ measurement	8*	For each variable of interest, give sources of data and details of methods of assessment (measurement). Describe comparability of assessment methods if there is more than one group.	
Bias	9	Describe any efforts to address potential sources of bias.	
Study size	10	Explain how the study size was arrived at.	
Quantitative variables	11	Explain how quantitative variables were handled in the analyses. If applicable, describe which groupings were chosen and why.	
Statistical methods	12	(a) Describe all statistical methods, including those used to control for confounding.	
		(b) Describe any methods used to examine subgroups and interactions.	
		(c) Explain how missing data were addressed.	
		(d) *Cohort study* – If applicable, explain how loss to follow-up was addressed. *Case-control study* – If applicable, explain how matching of cases and controls was addressed. *Cross-sectional study* – If applicable, describe analytical methods, taking account of sampling strategy.	
		(e) Describe any sensitivity analyses.	
Results			
Participants	13*	(a) Report numbers of individuals at each stage of study; for example, numbers potentially eligible, examined for eligibility, confirmed eligible, included in the study, completing follow-up and analysed.	
		(b) Give reasons for non-participation at each stage.	
		(c) Consider use of a flow diagram.	

	Item no.	Recommendation	Page no.
Descriptive data	14*	(a) Give characteristics of study participants (for example, demographic, clinical, social) and information on exposures and potential confounders.	
		(b) Indicate number of participants with missing data for each variable of interest.	
		(c) *Cohort study* – Summarise follow-up time (for example, average and total amount).	
Outcome data	15*	*Cohort study* – Report numbers of outcome events or summary measures over time.	
		Case-control study – Report numbers in each exposure category, or summary measures of exposure.	
		Cross-sectional study – Report numbers of outcome events or summary measures.	
Main results	16	(a) Give unadjusted estimates and, if applicable, confounder-adjusted estimates and their precision (for example, 95% **confidence interval**). Make clear which confounders were adjusted for and why they were included.	
		(b) Report category boundaries when continuous variables were categorised.	
		(c) If relevant, consider translating estimates of relative risk into absolute risk for a meaningful time period.	
Other analyses	17	Report other analyses done; for example, analyses of subgroups and interactions, and sensitivity analyses.	
Discussion			
Key results	18	Summarise key results with reference to study objectives.	
Limitations	19	Discuss limitations of the study, taking into account sources of potential bias or imprecision. Discuss both direction and magnitude of any potential bias.	

(*continued*)

Box 4.4 STROBE and RECORD Reporting Criteria (*continued*)

	Item no.	Recommendation	Page no.
Interpretation	20	Give a cautious overall interpretation of results, considering objectives, limitations, multiplicity of analyses, results from similar studies and other relevant evidence.	
Generalisability	21	Discuss the generalisability (external validity) of the study results.	
Other information			
Funding	22	Give the source of funding and the role of the funders for the present study and, if applicable, for the original study on which the present article is based.	

*Give information separately for cases and controls in case-control studies and, if applicable, for exposed and unexposed groups in cohort and cross-sectional studies.

Source: Vandenbroucke et al. (2007).

RECORD Reporting Criteria

	Item no.	STROBE items	Location in manuscript where items are reported	RECORD items	Location in manuscript where items are reported
Title and abstract					
	1	(a) Indicate the study's design with a commonly used term in the title or the abstract (b) Provide in the abstract an informative and balanced summary of what was done and what was found.		RECORD 1.1: The type of data used should be specified in the title or abstract. When possible, the name of the databases used should be included. RECORD 1.2: If applicable, the geographic region and	

	Item no.	STROBE items	Location in manuscript where items are reported	RECORD items	Location in manuscript where items are reported
				timeframe within which the study took place should be reported in the title or abstract.	
				RECORD 1.3: If linkage between databases was conducted for the study, this should be clearly stated in the title or abstract.	
Introduction					
Background rationale	2	Explain the scientific background and rationale for the investigation being reported.			
Objectives	3	State specific objectives, including any prespecified hypotheses.			
Methods					
Study design	4	Present key elements of study design early in the paper.			

(continued)

Box 4.4 STROBE and RECORD Reporting Criteria (*continued*)

	Item no.	STROBE items	Location in manuscript where items are reported	RECORD items	Location in manuscript where items are reported
Setting	5	Describe the setting, locations and relevant dates, including periods of recruitment, exposure, follow-up and data collection.			
Participants	6	(a) *Cohort study* – Give the eligibility criteria, and the sources and methods of selection of participants. Describe methods of follow-up. *Case-control study* – Give the eligibility criteria, and the sources and methods of case ascertainment and control selection. Give the rationale for the choice of cases and controls. *Cross-sectional study* – Give the eligibility criteria, and the sources and		RECORD 6.1: The methods of study population selection (such as codes or algorithms used to identify subjects) should be listed in detail. If this is not possible, an explanation should be provided. RECORD 6.2: Any validation studies of the codes or algorithms used to select the population should be referenced. If validation was conducted for this study and not published elsewhere, detailed	

	Item no.	STROBE items	Location in manuscript where items are reported	RECORD items	Location in manuscript where items are reported
		methods of selection of participants. (b) *Cohort study* – For matched studies, give matching criteria and number of exposed and unexposed. *Case-control study* – For matched studies, give matching criteria and the number of controls per case.		methods and results should be provided. RECORD 6.3: If the study involved linkage of databases, consider use of a flow diagram or other graphical display to demonstrate the data linkage process, including the number of individuals with linked data at each stage.	
Variables	7	Clearly define all outcomes, exposures, predictors, potential confounders and effect modifiers. Give diagnostic criteria, if applicable.		RECORD 7.1: A complete list of codes and algorithms used to classify exposures, outcomes, confounders and effect modifiers should be provided. If these cannot be reported, an explanation should be provided.	

(continued)

Box 4.4 STROBE and RECORD Reporting Criteria (*continued*)

	Item no.	STROBE items	Location in manuscript where items are reported	RECORD items	Location in manuscript where items are reported
Data sources/ measurement	8	For each variable of interest, give sources of data and details of methods of assessment (measurement). Describe comparability of assessment methods if there is more than one group.			
Bias	9	Describe any efforts to address potential sources of bias.			
Study size	10	Explain how the study size was arrived at.			
Quantitative variables	11	Explain how quantitative variables were handled in the analyses. If applicable, describe which groupings were chosen, and why.			
Statistical methods	12	(a) Describe all statistical methods, including those used to control for confounding.			

	Item no.	STROBE items	Location in manuscript where items are reported	RECORD items	Location in manuscript where items are reported
		(b) Describe any methods used to examine subgroups and interactions.			
		(c) Explain how missing data were addressed.			
		(d) *Cohort study* – If applicable, explain how loss to follow-up was addressed.			
		Case-control study – If applicable, explain how matching of cases and controls was addressed.			
		Cross-sectional study – If applicable, describe analytical methods, taking account of sampling strategy.			
		(e) Describe any sensitivity analyses.			
Data access and cleaning methods		..		RECORD 12.1: Authors should describe the extent to which	

(*continued*)

Box 4.4 STROBE and RECORD Reporting Criteria (*continued*)

	Item no.	STROBE items	Location in manuscript where items are reported	RECORD items	Location in manuscript where items are reported
				the investigators had access to the database population used to create the study population. RECORD 12.2: Authors should provide information on the data cleaning methods used in the study.	
Linkage		..		RECORD 12.3: State whether the study included person-level, institutional-level or other data linkage across two or more databases. The methods of linkage and methods of linkage quality evaluation should be provided.	
Results					
Participants	13	(a) Report the numbers of individuals at each stage of the study.		RECORD 13.1: Describe in detail the selection of the persons	

	Item no.	STROBE items	Location in manuscript where items are reported	RECORD items	Location in manuscript where items are reported
		(for example, numbers potentially eligible, examined for eligibility, confirmed eligible, included in the study, completing follow-up and analysed). (b) Give reasons for non-participation at each stage (c) Consider use of a flow diagram.		included in the study (i.e. study population selection), including filtering based on data quality, data availability and linkage. The selection of included persons can be described in the text and/or by means of the study flow diagram.	
Descriptive data	14	(a) Give characteristics of study participants (for example, demographic, clinical, social) and information on exposures and potential confounders. (b) Indicate the number of participants with missing data for each variable of interest.			

(continued)

Box 4.4 STROBE and RECORD Reporting Criteria (*continued*)

	Item no.	STROBE items	Location in manuscript where items are reported	RECORD items	Location in manuscript where items are reported
		(c) *Cohort study* – summarise follow-up time (for example, average and total amount).			
Outcome data	15	*Cohort study* – Report numbers of outcome events or summary measures over time. *Case-control study* – Report numbers in each exposure category, or summary measures of exposure. *Cross-sectional study* – Report numbers of outcome events or summary measures.			
Main results	16	(a) Give unadjusted estimates and, if applicable, confounder-adjusted estimates and their precision (for example, 95% confidence interval). Make.			

	Item no.	STROBE items	Location in manuscript where items are reported	RECORD items	Location in manuscript where items are reported
		clear which confounders were adjusted for and why they were included.			
		(b) Report category boundaries when continuous variables were categorised.			
		(c) If relevant, consider translating estimates of relative risk into absolute risk for a meaningful time period.			
Other analyses	17	Report other analyses done; for example, analyses of subgroups and interactions, and sensitivity analyses.			
Discussion					
Key results	18	Summarise key results with reference to study objectives.			

(continued)

Box 4.4 STROBE and RECORD Reporting Criteria (*continued*)

	Item no.	STROBE items	Location in manuscript where items are reported	RECORD items	Location in manuscript where items are reported
Limitations	19	Discuss limitations of the study, taking into account sources of potential bias or imprecision. Discuss both direction and magnitude of any potential bias.		RECORD 19.1: Discuss the implications of using data that were not created or collected to answer the specific research question(s). Include discussion of misclassification bias, unmeasured confounding, missing data and changing eligibility over time, as they pertain to the study being reported.	
Interpretation	20	Give a cautious overall interpretation of results, considering objectives, limitations, multiplicity of analyses, results from similar studies and other relevant evidence.			

	Item no.	STROBE items	Location in manuscript where items are reported	RECORD items	Location in manuscript where items are reported
Generali-sability	21	Discuss the generalisability (external validity) of the study results.			
Other information					
Funding	22	Give the source of funding and the role of the funders for the present study and, if applicable, for the original study on which the present article is based.			
Accessibility of **protocol**, raw data and programming code		..		RECORD 22.1: Authors should provide information on how to access any supplemental information such as the study protocol, raw data or programming code.	

Source: Benchimol et al. (2015).

Summary

Observational studies are common in prehospital and emergency medicine research, and can provide valuable information on incidence, prevalence and associations between exposures and outcomes, particularly where the research question cannot be addressed through a randomised trial. Observational studies also play a valuable role in providing cost-effective, 'real-world' evidence; monitoring for longer term outcomes or side effects that present beyond trial follow-up periods; and providing preliminary data to inform trials. However, observational studies have several limitations, are prone to confounding and bias and cannot generally be used to provide evidence of causal relationships. Results should therefore be reported and interpreted with this in mind.

Further Reading

Black, N. 1996. Why we need observational studies to evaluate the effectiveness of health care. *BMJ*, 312, 1215–1218.

Gershon, A. S. et al. 2018. Clinical knowledge from observational studies. Everything you wanted to know but were afraid to ask. *American Journal of Respiratory and Critical Care Medicine*, 198, 859–867.

Hackshaw, A. 2014. *A Concise Guide to Observational Studies in Healthcare*. BMJ Books, John Wiley and Sons, Ltd, New Jersey.

Mann, C. J. 2003. Observational research methods. Research design II: Cohort, cross sectional, and case-control studies. *Emergency Medicine Journal*, 20, 54–60.

Schulz, K. and Grimes, D. 2019. *Essential Concepts in Clinical Research: Randomised Controlled Trials and Observational Epidemiology*. Elsevier, Amsterdam.

Spiegelhalter, D. 2020. *The Art of Statistics: Learning from Data*. Pelican Books, London.

Venkatesh, A. K. et al. 2017. Systematic review of emergency medicine clinical practice guidelines: Implications for research and policy. *PLoS One*, 12, e0178456.

References

Andersen, L. W. and Kurth, T. 2018. Propensity scores – A brief introduction for resuscitation researchers. *Resuscitation*, 125, 66–69.

Andersen, L. W., Grossestreuer, A. V. and Donnino, M. W. 2018. "Resuscitation time bias" – A unique challenge for observational cardiac arrest research. *Resuscitation*, 125, 79–82.

Badcock, D. et al. 2005. The quality of medical record review studies in the international emergency medicine literature. *Annals of Emergency Medicine*, 45, 444–447.

Benchimol, E. I. et al. 2015. RECORD Working Committee. The REporting of studies Conducted using Observational Routinely-collected health Data (RECORD) statement. *PLoS Medicine*, 12, e1001885.

Benchimol, E. I. et al. 2020. Retraction of COVID-19 pharmacoepidemiology research could have been avoided by effective use of reporting guidelines. *Clinical Epidemiology*, 12, 1403–1420.

Bowman, L. et al. 2020. Understanding the use of observational and randomized data in cardiovascular medicine. *European Heart Journal*, 41, 2571–2578.

Busch, A. et al. 2016. Vascular type Ehlers-Danlos syndrome is associated with platelet dysfunction and low vitamin D serum concentration. *Orphanet Journal of Rare Diseases*, 11, 111.

Charlton, K., Limmer, M. and Moore, H. 2020. Intravenous versus oral paracetamol in a UK ambulance service: A case control study. *British Paramedic Journal*, 5, 1–6.

Cohen, A. T. et al. 2015. Why do we need observational studies of everyday patients in the real-life setting? *European Heart Journal Supplements*, 17, D2–D8.

Couper, K. et al. 2018. Patient, health service factors and variation in mortality following resuscitated out-of-hospital cardiac arrest in acute coronary syndrome: Analysis of the Myocardial Ischaemia National Audit Project. *Resuscitation*, 124, 49–57.

Dagan, N. et al. 2021. BNT162b2 mRNA Covid-19 vaccine in a nationwide mass vaccination setting. *The New England Journal of Medicine*, 384, 1412–1423.

Delgado-Rodríguez, M. and Llorca, J. 2004. Bias. *Journal of Epidemiology and Community Health*, 58, 635–641.

Dickson, J. M. et al. 2016. Cross-sectional study of the prehospital management of adult patients with a suspected seizure (EPIC1). *BMJ Open*, 6, e010573.

Fanaroff, A. C., Califf, R. M. and Windecker, S. 2019. Levels of evidence supporting American College of Cardiology/American Heart Association and European Society of Cardiology guidelines, 2008–2018. *JAMA*, 321, 1069 –1080.

Gavalova, L. et al. 2019. Use and impact of the prehospital 12-lead ECG in the primary PCI era (PHECG2): Protocol for a mixed-method study. *Open Heart*, 6, e001156.

Herrett, E. et al. 2013. Completeness and diagnostic validity of recording acute myocardial infarction events in primary care, hospital care, disease registry, and national mortality records: cohort study. *BMJ*, 346, f2350.

Hofmann, R. et al. 2017. DETO2X–SWEDEHEART Investigators. Oxygen therapy in suspected acute myocardial infarction. *The New England Journal of Medicine*, 377, 1240–1249.

Ji, C., Quinn, T. et al. 2018. Feasibility of data linkage in the PARAMEDIC trial: A cluster randomised trial of mechanical chest compression in out-of-hospital cardiac arrest. *BMJ Open*, 8, e021519.

Kaji, A. H., Schriger, D. and Green, S. 2014. Looking through the retrospectoscope: Reducing bias in emergency medicine chart review studies. *Annals of Emergency Medicine*, 64, 292–298.

Kohli, P. and Cannon, C. P. 2012. The importance of matching language to type of evidence: Avoiding the pitfalls of reporting outcomes data. *Clinical Cardiology*, 35, 714–717.

Latten, G. et al. 2020. How well are sepsis and a sense of urgency documented throughout the acute care chain in the Netherlands? A prospective, observational study. *BMJ Open*, 10, e036276.

Laudermilch, D. J. et al. 2010. Lack of emergency medical services documentation is associated with poor patient outcomes: A validation of audit filters for prehospital trauma care. *Journal of the American College of Surgeons*, 210, 220–227.

Lee, K. J. et al. 2021. STRATOS initiative. Framework for the treatment and reporting of missing data in observational studies: The Treatment and Reporting of Missing data in Observational Studies framework. *Journal of Clinical Epidemiology*, 134, 79–88.

McHugh, M. L. 2012. Interrater reliability: The kappa statistic. *Biochemia Medica (Zagreb)*, 22, 276–282.

McLachlan, S. et al. 2021. Scoping the demand for night operation of Essex and Herts Air Ambulance: A prospective observational study. *Air Medical Journal*, 40, 28–35.

McNamara, R. L. 2010. Cardiovascular registry research comes of age. *Heart*, 96, 908–910.

Merchant, R. M., Topjian, A. A. and Panchal, A. R. 2020. Part 1: Executive summary: 2020 American Heart Association guidelines for cardiopulmonary resuscitation and emergency cardiovascular care. *Circulation*, 142, S337–S357.

Morshed, S., Tornetta, P. 3rd and Bhandari, M. 2009. Analysis of observational studies: A guide to understanding statistical methods. *Journal of Bone and Joint Surgery*, 91, 50–60.

O'Neill, S., Graham, B. and Ennis, E. 2019. Emergency department and hospital care prior to suicide: A population based case control study. *Journal of Affective Disorders*, 249, 366–370.

Patridge, E. and Bardyn, T. 2018. Research Electronic Data Capture (REDCap). *Journal of the Medical Library Association*, 106, 142–144.

Porter, A. et al. 2008. "Covering our backs": Ambulance crews' attitudes towards clinical documentation when emergency (999) patients are not conveyed to hospital. *Emergency Medicine Journal*, 25, 292–295.

Porter, A. et al. 2020. Electronic health records in ambulances: The ERA multiple-methods study. *Health Services and Delivery Research*, 8, 10.

Puymirat, E., Battler, A. and Birkhead, J. 2013. Euro Heart Survey 2009 Snapshot: Regional variations in presentation and management of patients with AMI in 47 countries. *European Heart Journal. Acute Cardiovascular Care*, 2, 359–370.

Quinn, T. et al. 2014. Myocardial Ischaemia National Audit Project (MINAP) steering group. Effects of prehospital 12-lead ECG on processes of care and mortality in acute coronary syndrome: A linked cohort study from the Myocardial Ischaemia National Audit Project. *Heart*, 100, 944–950.

Sakurai, A. et al. 2019. Confirmed cardiac output on emergency medical services arrival as confounding by indication: An observational study of prehospital airway management in patients with out-of-hospital cardiac arrest. *Emergency Medicine Journal*, 36, 410–415.

Schulz, K. F. and Grimes, D. A. 2019. *Essential Concepts in Clinical Research: Randomised Controlled Trials and Observational Epidemiology*. London, Elsevier.

Siriwardena, A. N. et al. 2019. Patient and clinician factors associated with prehospital pain treatment and outcomes: Cross sectional study. *The American Journal of Emergency Medicine*, 37, 266–271.

Six, A. J. et al. 2013. The HEART score for the assessment of patients with chest pain in the emergency department: A multinational validation study. *Critical Pathways in Cardiology*, 12, 121–126.

Smith, J. et al. 2020. Evolution of methodology and reporting of emergency medicine quantitative research over a 20-year period. *Emergency Medicine Journal*, 37, 324–329.

Sorgentone, S. et al. 2021. A large food-borne outbreak of campylobacteriosis in kindergartens and primary schools in Pescara, Italy, May–June 2018. *Journal of Medical Microbiology*, 70.

Spiegelhalter, D. 2019. *The Art of Statistics: Learning from Data*. Pelican Books, London.

Staff, T. and Søvik, S. 2011. A retrospective quality assessment of prehospital emergency medical documentation in motor vehicle accidents in south-eastern Norway. *Scandinavian Journal of Trauma, Resuscitation and Emergency Medicine*, 19, 20.

Stopyra, J., Snavely, A. and Smith, L. 2020. Prehospital use of a modified HEART Pathway and point-of-care troponin to predict cardiovascular events. *PLoS One*, 15, e0239460.

Sultanian, P. et al. 2021. Cardiac arrest in COVID-19: Characteristics and outcomes of in- and out-of-hospital cardiac arrest. A report from the Swedish Registry for Cardiopulmonary Resuscitation. *European Heart Journal*, 42, 1094–1106.

Vandenbroucke, J. P. et al. 2007. Strengthening the Reporting of Observational Studies in Epidemiology (STROBE): Explanation and elaboration. *PLoS Medicine*, 4.

von Elm, E. et al. 2014. STROBE initiative. The Strengthening the Reporting of Observational Studies in Epidemiology (STROBE) statement: Guidelines for reporting observational studies. *International Journal of Surgery*, 12, 1495–1499.

Voss, S. et al. 2018. How do people with dementia use the ambulance service? A retrospective study in England: The HOMEWARD project. *BMJ Open*, 8, e022549.

Worster, A. et al. 2005. Reassessing the methods of medical record review studies in emergency medicine research. *Annals of Emergency Medicine*, 45, 448–451.

Chapter 5

Experimental and Quasi-experimental Designs

Gavin Perkins, Chen Ji and Mike Smyth

Chapter Objectives

This chapter will cover:

- The different types of quasi-experimental and experimental design
- Examples of quasi-experimental and experimental designs used in prehospital research
- The design features of quasi-experimental and experimental studies
- The advantages and disadvantages of these different study designs
- The role of checklists when designing and reporting study findings

---

Introduction

As described in the previous chapter, observational studies play an important role in examining associations between particular treatments and health **outcomes**. However, due to the risks of **bias** and **confounding**, they are unable to determine cause and effect and should be considered as hypothesis generating.

Quasi-experimental studies are non-randomised, controlled studies designed to evaluate the effects of specific interventions/treatments on health outcomes. Although these designs have the potential to reduce bias and confounding, they cannot eliminate them completely.

Randomised controlled trials aim to overcome some of these limitations by allocating individuals by chance to an intervention or control. The outcomes of interest are then compared between the two groups at the end of the trial. A well-conducted randomised controlled trial provides the most reliable information about the effectiveness or otherwise of an intervention, hence its inclusion near the top of the pyramid for evidence-based medicine (see **Chapter 1, Figure 1.1**).

Quasi-experimental Designs

Quasi-experimental evaluations, also referred to as non-randomised studies, are often used in prehospital care **research** (Bärnighausen et al., 2017; Mann, 2003;

Nichol and Huszti, 2007). Outcomes are analysed by comparing two groups by the treatments they received. There are three main types of quasi-experimental designs used in prehospital research: 1) **before-and-after studies**, 2) **interrupted time series** and 3) **propensity score matching**. Quasi-experimental studies are simpler and less costly to perform than the gold standard of randomised controlled trials. They can also overcome some of the practical and ethical challenges encountered when trying to conduct a randomised evaluation. Other advantages include increasing the **generalisability** of findings, as the characteristics of participants **enrolled** typically resemble the population of interest. Quasi-experimental studies are usually pragmatic in that they test the effectiveness (real-world effects) of an intervention, unlike in the controlled conditions seen in some randomised trials. Quasi-experimental studies can be undertaken prospectively or retrospectively, allowing evaluation of changes to health policy and clinical guidelines (Schweizer et al., 2016).

However, quasi-experimental study designs are susceptible to bias and confounding (see **Box 5.1**). This may lead to non-random differences in important prognostic factors between intervention and control groups, which make it difficult to demonstrate a cause–effect or causal relationship between the intervention and outcome. The findings must therefore be interpreted with caution when assigning causality to the intervention.

There are a number of different sources of bias in prehospital research. **Selection bias** can occur due to systematic differences between the group who receive the intervention and the baseline/control group, for example, in age, sex, ethnicity or socio-economic status. Other examples of selection bias seen commonly in observational cardiac arrest studies include immortal time bias and resuscitation time bias (Andersen et al., 2018). If one considers an observational study of targeted temperature management (TTM) following return of spontaneous circulation, patients who die before they receive TTM will by default be included in the 'control' group as they did not survive long enough to receive TTM. This will bias in favour of those who were alive long enough to receive TTM. The converse occurs in resuscitation time bias – which leads to the biased association between interventions given during cardiac arrest. As the chances of survival reduce the longer someone is in cardiac arrest, interventions given later in the treatment pathway (for example, intubation, drug administration) bias towards those interventions appearing to

---

Box 5.1 Bias and Confounding

Bias: Any systematic error in a study that results in an incorrect estimate of the true effect of an exposure on the outcome of interest.

Confounding: Distortion of the association between an exposure and outcome of interest by an extraneous third variable called a **confounder**.

be associated with worse outcomes. Whilst careful control of eligibility criteria or statistical modelling, which includes adjustment for the time someone is 'at risk' of a particular intervention, can minimise the impact of these biases, many studies fail to adequately control for them.

Other factors that threaten the **internal validity** of quasi-experimental studies include changes occurring due to the passage of time unrelated to the intervention being evaluated. This is known as maturation bias if it relates to changes in the study subject; for example, CPR given in the early or late stages of cardiac arrest, and temporal bias if it relates to changes to clinical practice such as new guidelines being published. A Hawthorne effect (where behaviours change due to an awareness that performance is being monitored) can be problematic if data from the control phase are collected retrospectively but results from the intervention phase occur after those participating in the research become aware of the study objectives (Handley et al., 2018; Schweizer et al., 2016).

Other limitations can include problems with data quality (particularly if data are collected routinely or retrospectively as part of the clinical record) or if definition or measurement tools for the outcome of interest change over time. For example, the change in diagnosis of cardiac arrest from absent breathing with no pulse, to absent or abnormal breathing (without a requirement for pulse palpation) may have changed the characteristics of people identified as having sustained a cardiac arrest (Cummins and Hazinski, 2000). Regression to the mean is a statistical phenomenon whereby the natural variation in data appears to reflect an important difference, when in reality there is no important difference. It commonly occurs when an outlier (unusually small or large measurement) is followed by a measurement closer to the mean (average). For example, heavy rain may adversely impact ambulance response times for a short period. A small number of prolonged response times will make the mean (average) response time for that particular 24-hour period appear to be worse, but such a blip in response times does not necessarily mean performance of the ambulance service is declining. Once road conditions improve, it is likely that mean ambulance response times will improve too. Such natural variations in data can become a problem if the variation occurs between the control or intervention phases, creating the potential to misinterpret differences in performance. Such natural variation becomes a problem when it occurs between the control or intervention phase during before-and-after and time-series studies.

Examples of Prehospital Quasi-experimental Designs

Before-and-after studies

In before-and-after studies, the dependent variable (outcome of interest) is measured before the intervention is implemented (control phase) and after it has been implemented (intervention phase). If there is a difference in the dependent variable between the control phase and intervention phase then one plausible explanation is that the intervention led to the observed change. See **Box 5.2** for a before-and-after study example.

> ## Box 5.2 Case Study: Ontario Prehospital Advanced Life Support Study (Stiell et al., 2004)
>
> The Ontario Prehospital Advanced Life Support (OPALS) study evaluated the controlled introduction of advanced life support interventions (advanced airways and drugs) across 17 cities in Ontario, Canada. The study comprised two phases – a rapid defibrillation phase (control) where rapid defibrillation was optimised, followed by an intervention phase where paramedics with advanced training (airway and drug administration) were introduced into the healthcare system. The study enrolled 1,391 patients in the rapid defibrillation (control) phase and 4,247 in the advanced life support (intervention) phase. It found that the advanced life support phase improved the rates of return of spontaneous circulation from 12.9% to 18%, the proportion of patients admitted to hospital (10.9% versus 14.6%), but did not affect survival to hospital discharge (5.0% versus 5.1%) or cerebral performance category (level 1) amongst survivors (78.3% versus 66.8%).

Interrupted Time Series

Interrupted time-series analyses take several measurements before and after the implementation of an intervention in order to determine the intervention's effect over a period of time. Analyses typically look for a step change in the outcome before and after the implementation of the intervention or a change in the slope/trajectory of the outcome. This is known as the interruption. See **Box 5.3** for an example of interrupted time-series analysis.

Propensity Score Matching

Propensity score matching is a statistical technique that artificially creates control and intervention groups, from within a population of patients, some of whom received an intervention and others who did not. It requires large sample sizes and complete information about the covariates that will be used for matching. The technique seeks to match each patient who received an intervention with one or more patients, who have similar characteristics, but who did not receive the intervention. By matching patients with similar baseline characteristics who did and did not receive the intervention, it creates intervention and control groups and enables comparison between these groups. See **Box 5.4** for an example of propensity score matching.

Experimental Designs (Randomised Controlled Trials)

The US National Institute of Health defines a clinical trial as a 'research study in which one or more human subjects are prospectively assigned to one or more interventions (which may include placebo or other control) to evaluate the effects of those interventions on health-related biomedical or behavioural outcomes' (National Institute for Health, n.d.). Well-conducted randomised controlled trials are considered

Box 5.3 Case Study: Introduction of Major Trauma Systems to the NHS (Moran et al., 2018)

Major trauma networks were introduced in the NHS in England in 2012, which enabled ambulances to bypass local hospitals and convey patients to one of 27 newly designated Major Trauma Centres. The Trauma Audit and Research Network (TARN) undertook a longitudinal analysis of the outcomes of patients who sustained major trauma between 2008 and 2017. An interrupted time-series analysis was used to look for evidence of a step change in outcomes as well as differences over time.

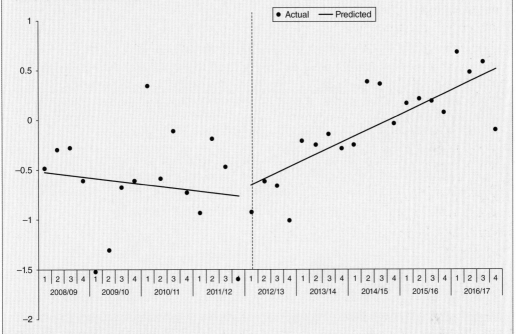

Source: Moran et al. (2018).

The interrupted time-series analysis presents the excess survival rate per 100 patients (y axis) against time (x axis). There was no difference in survival outcomes in the four years preceding the roll-out of trauma networks (left side of diagram). After implementation (Quarter 1 2012/13), there was a statistically significant positive change in the slope, indicating an increase in the number of survivors after implementation of major trauma networks.

the gold standard for the evaluation of healthcare interventions as they reduce the risk of bias through balancing the characteristics of participants (both measured and unmeasured) between the groups. Any differences in outcomes can be attributed to the trial intervention. See **Box 5.5** for the key components of a randomised controlled trial.

Box 5.4 Case Study: Prehospital Adrenaline Use and Survival Amongst Patients With Out-of-Hospital Cardiac Arrest (Hagihara et al., 2012)

Adrenaline has been used for many years as a treatment for cardiac arrest. Its use became established in prehospital care as observational studies showed that it is highly effective at restarting the heart, but there was less evidence of it having beneficial effects on long-term outcomes. The OPALS study reviewed above failed to show benefit for adrenaline on long-term survival or favourable neurological outcome.

Japan example

Adrenaline was introduced into prehospital care in Japan in April 2006. The study authors compared the outcomes of those who received adrenaline with those who did not receive adrenaline. To minimise the potential for confounding and selection bias the authors developed a propensity score for each participant based on characteristics that were known to be associated with outcome (for example, age, bystander CPR, bystander defibrillation, initial rhythm). Participants with similar propensity scores were compared between the intervention and the control groups.

The first analysis of these data by Hagihara et al. (2012) reported that adrenaline was associated with a decreased chance of survival and good functional outcomes at one month after the event. However, this analysis did not take into account the influence of resuscitation bias as described above. A further analysis of the same database by Nakahara et al. (2013), which included matching for the time of drug administration, reported that adrenaline improved long-term survival, albeit with minimal effect on favourable neurological outcomes. These divergent findings highlight the importance of ensuring the inclusion of important potential confounding variables in analyses.

Box 5.5 Key Components of Randomised Controlled Trials

- They have a clearly defined research question.
- They have a trial **protocol** that describes the rationale, intervention and all related trial procedures and follow-up plans.
- There is random allocation between intervention groups.
- Where possible, patients and/or those conducting the trial and assessing outcomes are masked to treatment allocation.
- All intervention groups are treated the same except for the experimental treatment.
- Analysis occurs on the basis of intention to treat (that is, analysed within the group they were allocated).
- They assess differences between interventions according to pre-defined outcomes.

Although there are many advantages of randomised controlled trials, they face limitations as well. A key limitation of randomised controlled trials can be the complexity and cost to set up and deliver them. This can be mitigated at least in part by embedding trial processes in routine clinical practice and making use of existing data collection tools where possible. Ethical problems can be encountered during the conduct of clinical trials if evidence becomes available that one treatment is better than another, that is, there is a loss of clinical **equipoise**, which can lead to early discontinuation of a trial. Despite these challenges, clinical trials play a major role in providing reliable evidence to guide clinical practice.

Defining the Research Question

The first step in designing a randomised controlled trial is to define the research question using the Population, Intervention, Comparator, Outcome (**PICO**) format.

- *Population*: Define the characteristics of participants who will be enrolled in the trial.

- *Intervention*: Describe the trial intervention, which may be a drug, device or other intervention (for example, call handler instructions, post-resuscitation debriefing).

- *Comparator*: Depending on the study design, this could be a placebo or standard care (treatment as usual).

- *Outcome:* Describe the outcomes of interest. The primary outcome is the main / most important outcome and the one which will determine the size of the trial. Secondary outcomes are other outcomes of importance and can be patient focused (such as pain score), survival, resource use (such as length of hospital stay), health-related quality of life or economic outcomes. Core outcome sets can be used to promote consistency in outcomes reported by different trials. This helps to facilitate pooling trial results in meta-analyses. The Core Outcome Set for Cardiac Arrest (COSCA) is one example (Haywood et al., 2018). Examples of the PICO framework are shown in **Table 5.1**.

Terminology and Development Pathways

The development pathway for drugs typically involves four phases. **Phase 1 studies** (sometimes called first-in-human studies) seek to assess safety and tolerability in healthy volunteers. **Phase 2 studies** (sometimes called efficacy trials) aim to demonstrate proof of concept that a drug has a therapeutic effect and to identify the optimal dose. They typically enrol 100–500 patients. **Phase 3 studies** (sometimes called effectiveness or confirmatory trials) set out to confirm the safety and effectiveness of the drug in larger numbers of patients (1,000–5,000). **Phase 4 studies** focus on long-term surveillance of safety and real-life performance of the drugs in practice. They can also explore additional indications where the drug may be effective.

Table 5.1 – Examples of PICO questions for UK prehospital trials.

	PARAMEDIC (Perkins et al., 2015)	PARAMEDIC2 (Perkins et al., 2018)	RePHILL (Smith et al., 2018)
Population	Adults with OHCA	Adults with OHCA	Adults with hypotension due to traumatic haemorrhage
Intervention	Mechanical CPR	Adrenaline 1 milligram	Packed red blood cells and lyophi-lised plasma
Comparator	Standard CPR	0.9% saline	0.9% saline
Outcome	30-day survival	30-day survival	Episode mortality and lactate clearance

Alternative terms used to describe clinical trials can include **feasibility**/pilot and explanatory/pragmatic trials. Feasibility studies are undertaken to determine if a piece of research is feasible, not to answer a specific clinical question – in other words, they ask if the study can be done. Feasibility studies usually focus on recruitment, **randomisation**, follow-up rates and data completeness. They can also be used to estimate the event rates or other important parameters that are needed to calculate the sample size. **Pilot studies** are a version of the main study that is run in miniature to test whether the components of the main study can all work together. They are focused on the processes of the main study, for example, to ensure that recruitment, randomisation, treatment and follow-up assessments all run smoothly (Eldridge et al., 2016). Pilot studies can be internal (data obtained form part of the analysis for the main trial) or external (data are analysed separately from the main trial) (National Institute for Health Research, 2019). An explanatory trial is the term used when a treatment is tested under optimal conditions, as is typically seen in a phase 2 trial. Adherence to the protocol is strictly monitored, as is follow-up for the trial outcomes. Pragmatic trials, by contrast, test a treatment under real-world conditions. They seek to determine whether a treatment works in clinical practice, with limited supervision/oversight/control by the study investigators (Sedgwick, 2014).

Trials in prehospital care are usually designed to test if one treatment is better than other treatments or standard care. These trials are called superiority trials. Other, less-common designs are equivalence trials (which set out to see if two treatments deliver equivalent results) and non-inferiority trials (one treatment is no worse than the other treatment).

Routemap

The National Institute for Health Research has produced a Clinical Trials Toolkit, which outlines the various stages involved in setting up and running a Clinical Trial of an Investigational Medicinal Product (CTIMP). Although designed specifically for trials testing drugs, it serves as a useful framework for the steps involved in trials investigating interventions other than drugs. See **Figure 5.1** for the Clinical Trials Toolkit Routemap.

Trial Protocol

A trial protocol is a prerequisite for undertaking a randomised controlled trial. The protocol should describe the evidence base and rationale for the trial, the research question/hypothesis, the study design and how the trial will be conducted, analysed and reported. The Standard Protocol Items: Recommendations for Interventional Trials (SPIRIT) contain evidence-based recommendations for the core content of clinical trial protocols (Chan et al., 2013).

Randomisation

The process of randomly assigning a trial participant to the intervention or control group is called randomisation. It is the randomisation step that is essential for minimising the risk of bias, as if done correctly it should ensure that the participants in each arm of the trial have similar characteristics other than the intervention under evaluation.

There are two steps to randomisation – generating and then implementing the randomisation sequence. The generation of the randomised sequence (in other words, the order by which participants will be assigned to different treatments) is best done by a statistician or using a specialist computer program. The randomisation sequence should be developed based on a pre-defined ratio of intervention to control participants. In most trials, a 1:1 ratio is used (which means an equal number of participants are assigned to the intervention and control arms). Some trials have used an unequal sequence (such as the PARAMEDIC trial 1:2 ratio for intervention:control), as this was more cost efficient given the costs of the mechanical CPR device being studied (Dumville et al., 2006; Perkins et al., 2015). If randomisation were to occur in sequence – for example, ABABAB – the researcher could soon guess what the next treatment allocation would be, which risks selection bias. Block randomisation (where randomisation occurs in blocks of specific or variable sizes – for example, AABB, ABBABAAB – can reduce the risk of the researcher guessing the next randomised allocation. Additional steps to ensure that specific participant characteristics are evenly balanced include stratified randomisation and minimisation (see **Box 5.6**).

The second step of the randomisation process is implementation. A key requirement in the implementation step is to keep the allocation secret until the decision has been made to enrol a participant. If the randomised allocation were known by the researcher in advance, this could lead to selection bias (for example, the researcher

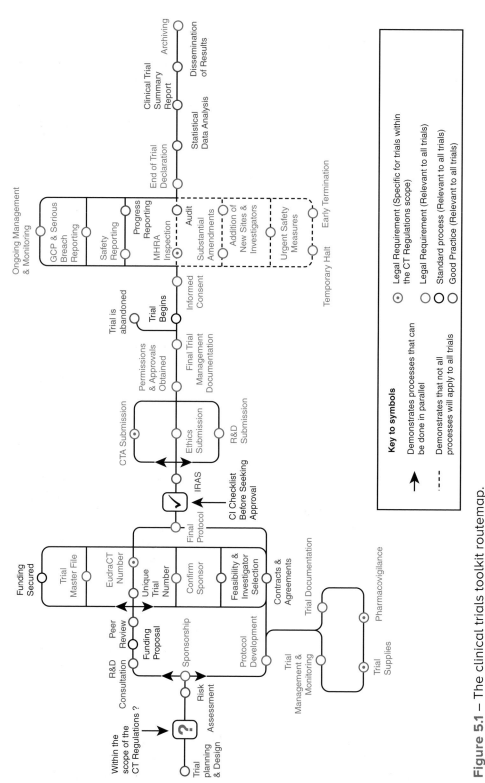

Figure 5.1 – The clinical trials toolkit routemap.

An interactive version is available at https://www.ct-toolkit.ac.uk/routemap/.

Abbreviations: R&D: Research and Development; CI: Chief Investigator; EudraCT: European Union Drug Regulating Authorities Clinical Trials Database; GCP: **Good Clinical Practice**; IRAS: Integrated Research Application System.

> ## Box 5.6 Stratified Randomisation and Minimisation Technique
>
> *Stratified randomisation*: Randomisation is performed within sub-groups of interest rather than on the population as a whole.
>
> *Minimisation technique*: The first participant is allocated a treatment at random. For subsequent participants, randomised allocation is based on which treatment would lead to better balance between the groups in the variables of interest.

may not enrol a participant if they do not think the intervention will work). Allocation concealment can be achieved in a number of ways. Secure, electronic randomisation (where randomisation occurs through a computer program or automated telephone service) is probably the most secure method. Other methods include the sequentially numbered treatment packs which are masked to prevent the person enrolling from knowing what the randomised treatment is. This approach was used in the ACUTE trial and PARAMEDIC2. Sealed envelopes have developed a bad reputation as a secure method for randomisation as they can be tampered with to reveal the treatment allocation (for example, opening the envelope in advance, shining the envelope against a bright light to reveal allocation), so they are generally best avoided (Torgerson and Roberts, 1999). Scratchcards have been used successfully as an alternative in prehospital research (Keen et al., 2018).

Study Designs

There are a number of different types of randomised trial designs. In the prehospital setting, the most commonly used approaches are parallel group design and cluster design trials. Other more complex designs such as factorial design or stepped wedge design have been used less frequently and some are unsuitable for prehospital research, for example, withdrawal trials (where participants are randomised to withdrawal of a specific treatment) or crossover trials (where participants receive the intervention and control treatments with a wash-out (treatment-free) period in between).

Parallel Group

This is a relatively common design in prehospital research (Fuller et al., 2021; Kudenchuk et al., 2016; Perkins et al., 2018). Participants are randomised individually to one of two treatment groups (see **Box 5.7**). The outcomes of interest are then compared between the two groups at the end of the trial.

Cluster

Cluster randomised trials are popular in prehospital care as they are often simpler to implement and set up than individually randomised trials and can reduce contamination. In cluster randomised trials, participants are randomised in groups

Box 5.7 Example: PARAMEDIC2 Trial was an Individual-patient Randomised Study (Perkins et al., 2018)

Consecutive patients were enrolled into the trial by opening sequentially numbered treatment packs. Half the packs contained adrenaline and half 0.9% saline. At the end of trial, the survival rates at 30 days were compared between the two groups.

8,014 participants

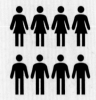

Treatment pack
Treatment pack
Treatment pack
Treatment pack
Treatment pack
Treatment pack
Treatment pack
Treatment pack

4,015 adrenaline arm

130 (3.2%) alive at 30 days

3,999 0.9% saline arm

94 (2.4%) alive at 30 days

Box 5.8 Example: PARAMEDIC Trial (Perkins et al., 2015)

In this trial, ambulance service vehicles (rapid response cars or ambulances) were randomised to either carry the mechanical CPR device (intervention arm) or to provide standard care (manual CPR). Patients received the treatment based on the allocation of the first ambulance vehicle to arrive on scene. To improve the cost efficiency of the trial, a randomisation ratio of 1:2 (intervention:control) was used as this reduced the number of intervention devices which needed to be supplied.

4,471 participants

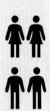

1,652 LUCAS arm

104 (6%) alive at 30 days

2,819 manual compression arm

193 (7%) alive at 30 days

(clusters) rather than individually (see **Box 5.8**). In other words, the treatment the person is randomised to receive is based on the group they fall in to rather than the individual person's characteristics. Clusters can be based on ambulance service or geographical areas (Hostler et al., 2011; Nichol et al., 2015; Snooks et al., 2017), ambulances (Perkins et al., 2015), pieces of equipment or the treating clinicians (Benger et al., 2018; Price et al., 2020). Disadvantages of cluster randomised trials are that they have less power and precision than individually randomised trials, which necessitates an increased sample size.

Factorial

Factorial trials examine the effects of two or more treatments simultaneously (see **Box 5.9**). In a 2 x 2 factorial design, participants are randomised to treatment A, treatment B, treatment A and B or control. This approach can be more efficient (it requires fewer participants to be recruited) than a multiple-arm individual patient randomised trial. A limitation of a factorial design approach is the possibility of an interaction between the two treatments (that is, the effect of one intervention depends on the presence or absence of another intervention) (Nichol and Huszti, 2007). A larger sample size is usually required to detect an interaction effect at the same power of main effects. Thus, the efficiency of the design could be compromised.

Box 5.9 Example: The Resuscitation Outcomes Consortium Prehospital Resuscitation Impedance Valve and Early Versus Delayed Analysis (ROC PRIMED) Trial

The ROC PRIMED trial randomised participants twice (Aufderheide et al., 2011; Stiell et al., 2011). The first randomisation allocated participants to an early or late rhythm analysis strategy. The second randomisation allocated participants to an active or sham impedance threshold device (ITD). The outcomes were then compared according to the groups they were randomised to. The trial is described as a partial factorial trial, as there were some differences in the inclusion criteria for each arm of the trial and not all EMS agencies participated in both trials. It nevertheless illustrates the general principles of a factorial design.

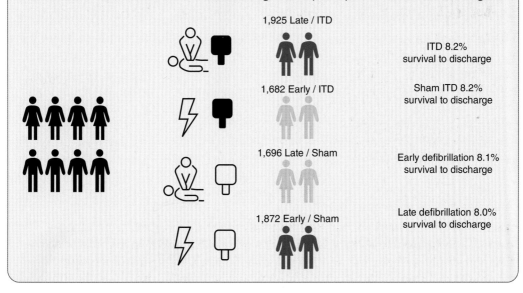

1,925 Late / ITD

1,682 Early / ITD

1,696 Late / Sham

1,872 Early / Sham

ITD 8.2% survival to discharge

Sham ITD 8.2% survival to discharge

Early defibrillation 8.1% survival to discharge

Late defibrillation 8.0% survival to discharge

Minimising the Risk of Bias

Clinical trials are designed to minimise the risk of bias, but not all trials are successful in managing bias effectively. The Cochrane collaboration classifies common sources of bias as falling into the following categories.

- *Selection bias* occurs when there are systematic differences in the baseline characteristics of the groups that are being compared or when participants are selected that are more or less likely to respond to the intervention. Selection bias can arise if allocation concealment is not successful, that is, the person enrolling participants to the trial is aware of the randomisation sequence before enrolment.

- *Performance bias* refers to systematic differences between treatment groups other than the intervention of interest. Steps to minimise the risk of performance bias include masking/blinding clinicians and participants to the randomised intervention.

- *Detection bias* describes the situation when systematic differences occur in the way outcomes are assessed between intervention arms. Withholding information about the randomised treatment arm from those assessing or reporting the outcomes will reduce detection bias.

- *Attrition bias* occurs when there are systematic differences in the number of participants who drop out from the trial, thus their outcome data are incomplete.

- *Reporting bias* occurs when researchers selectively report statistically significant differences rather than non-significant differences. Trial registration (such as clinicaltrials.gov) that records outcomes in advance of enrolling participants into a trial helps to minimise reporting bias.

Statistical Analysis

Involving a statistician and others with methodological expertise early in the design of a trial is essential to maximise the internal validity of the research. A key early step in designing a trial is to decide on the number of participants that need to be enrolled to answer the research question. Sample sizes are calculated according to the effect size (the minimum difference the trial wants to detect between treatment arms), power (the likelihood of a false negative result) and P value (the chance of a false positive trial result). All trials should have a statistical analysis plan that describes in advance how the trial outcomes will be analysed (Gamble et al., 2017). This is important for minimising selective analyses and reporting bias. Trial analyses are typically undertaken with and/or without adjustment for key participant baseline characteristics (Saquib et al., 2013).

As described above, most trials will analyse outcomes of interest on the basis of the intention-to-treat principle. This provides the best estimate of the real-world effectiveness of the intervention. An alternative strategy, per protocol, excludes participants with major protocol deviations, where key trial outcomes are unavailable or where the participant did not receive the intervention they were assigned to. Per protocol analyses provide information on how a treatment might work under optimal conditions.

Trial Conduct and Oversight

The term Good Clinical Practice (GCP) describes the ethical, scientific and practical standards by which all clinical research should be conducted. The purpose of GCP is to ensure that the rights, safety and well-being of participants in clinical research are protected and that the findings produced from research are reliable. Although there is a legal requirement to comply with GCP for Clinical Trials of Investigational Medicinal Products (CTIMP), it is best practice to ensure that all trials are conducted in accordance with the principles of GCP. Those leading and co-ordinating clinical trials are expected to have received training and to implement the principles of GCP during the conduct of the trial.

All clinical trials require a Sponsor. The Sponsor is the organisation that has overall responsibility for proportionate, effective arrangements being in place to set up, run and report the trial. The day-to-day operations of a clinical trial typically fall to a trial management group, comprising the chief investigator, trial manager and methodologists (statisticians and health economists), with input from research governance / quality assurance teams. Most large prehospital trials are run in collaboration with a Clinical Trials Unit. These larger studies are usually supervised by a Trial Steering Committee, a group of independent clinicians and methodologists who are responsible for the oversight of the trial. Data Monitoring Committees maintain close scrutiny on the accumulating data collected in the trial. The group are responsible for evaluating any interim analyses and may make recommendations to the Trial Steering Committee if there are any safety concerns or strong evidence for efficacy or futility. Both committees must ensure that the safety and well-being of participants are the study's first priority.

Clinical trials require review and approval by an independent Research Ethics Committee before they can commence. Additional approvals are required if the trial involves a drug (CTIMP) or unlicensed devices and for the processing of data if it is not possible to obtain consent from the participant or a legal representative.

CONSORT Reporting Guidelines

The Consolidated Standards of Reporting Trials (**CONSORT**) guidelines (Schulz et al., 2010) were developed as a framework to improve the reporting of randomised controlled trials. A key component of the standards is the CONSORT checklist, which identifies 25 items that should be included in reports of individually randomised, two-group parallel trials. Checklists for other trial designs, such as cluster or non-inferiority studies, have been developed and can be accessed

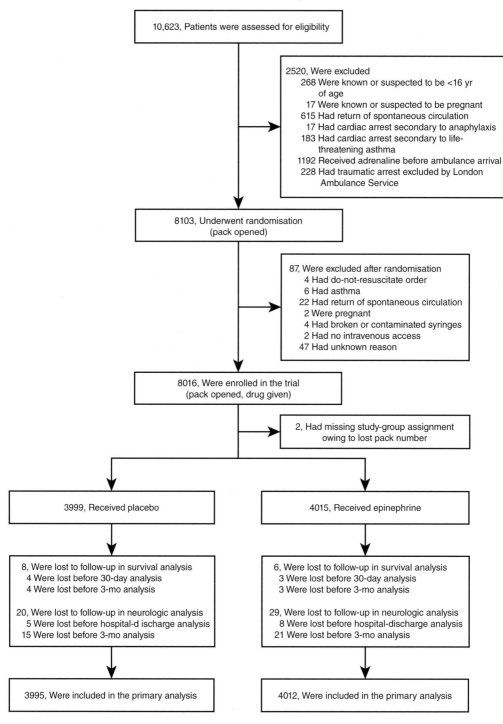

Figure 5.2 – CONSORT Flow Diagram for the PARAMEDIC2 Trial.

Source: Perkins et al. (2018).

at: http://www.consort-statement.org. Key components of the CONSORT requirements are the inclusion of a participant flow diagram that outlines the number of patients assessed for the trial, the reasons for any exclusions, how many were randomised and allocated to the intervention and control arms, how many received the randomised allocation and how many were lost to follow-up. The CONSORT flow diagram from PARAMEDIC2 is included as an example; see **Figure 5.2**.

Summary

Quasi-experimental (non-randomised) and experimental (randomised) studies seek to establish a cause-and-effect relationship between an outcome of interest (dependent variable) and intervention (independent variable). Quasi-experimental designs (which include before-and-after studies, time-series and propensity-matched scoring analyses) are often cheaper and simpler to organise than experimental designs but remain susceptible to bias and confounding. Experimental designs, by randomly assigning participants to intervention and control, seek to overcome the limitations of quasi-experimental studies. To achieve their full potential, it is important that randomised controlled trials are planned carefully and that due consideration is given to ensuring that the appropriate design is selected, that the trial is implemented effectively and that steps are taken to ensure the findings of the trial are transparently reported.

Further Reading

BMJ Epidemiology series. Chapter 9. Experimental studies. Available at: https://www.bmj.com/about-bmj/resources-readers/publications/epidemiology-uninitiated/13-further-reading.

Pocock, S. J. 2013. *Clinical Trials: A Practical Approach*. Wiley, Chichester.

Reichardt, C. S. 2019. *Quasi-Experimentation. A Guide to Design and Analysis 2019*. The Guilford Press, New York.

References

Andersen, L. W., Grossestreuer, A. V. and Donnino, M. W. 2018. "Resuscitation time bias": A unique challenge for observational cardiac arrest research. *Resuscitation*, 125, 79–82.

Aufderheide, T. P. et al. 2011. Standard cardiopulmonary resuscitation versus active compression-decompression cardiopulmonary resuscitation with augmentation of negative intrathoracic pressure for out-of-hospital cardiac arrest: A randomised trial. *Lancet*, 377, 301–311.

Bärnighausen, T. et al. 2017. Quasi-experimental study designs series—Paper 1: Introduction: Two historical lineages. *Journal Of Clinical Epidemiology*, 89, 4–11.

Benger, J. R. et al. 2018. Effect of a strategy of a supraglottic airway device vs tracheal intubation during out-of-hospital cardiac arrest on functional outcome: The Airways-2 randomized clinical trial. *JAMA*, 320, 779–791.

Chan, A. W. et al. 2013. SPIRIT 2013 explanation and elaboration: Guidance for protocols of clinical trials. *BMJ*, 346, E7586.

Cummins, R. O. and Hazinski, M. F. 2000. Guidelines based on fear of type ii (false-negative) errors. Why we dropped the pulse check for lay rescuers. *Resuscitation*, 46, 439–442.

Dumville, J. C. et al. 2006. The use of unequal randomisation ratios in clinical trials: A review. *Contemporary Clinical Trials*, 27, 1–12.

Eldridge, S. M. et al. 2016. Defining feasibility and pilot studies in preparation for randomised controlled trials: Development of a conceptual framework. *Plos One*, 11, E0150205.

Fuller, G. W. et al. 2021. Prehospital continuous positive airway pressure for acute respiratory failure: The acute feasibility RCT. *Health Technology Assessment*, 25, 1–92.

Gamble, C. et al. 2017. Guidelines for the content of statistical analysis plans in clinical trials. *JAMA*, 318, 2337–2343.

Hagihara, A. et al. 2012. Prehospital epinephrine use and survival among patients with out-of-hospital cardiac arrest. *JAMA*, 307, 1161–1168.

Handley, M. A. et al. 2018. Selecting and improving quasi-experimental designs in effectiveness and implementation research. *Annual Review of Public Health*, 39, 5–25.

Haywood, K. et al. 2018. COSCA (Core Outcome Set for Cardiac Arrest) in adults: An advisory statement from the International Liaison Committee on Resuscitation. *Resuscitation*, 127, 147–163.

Hostler, D. et al. 2011. Effect of real-time feedback during cardiopulmonary resuscitation outside hospital: Prospective, cluster-randomised trial. *BMJ*, 342.

Keen, L. et al. 2018. Use of scratchcards for allocation concealment in a prehospital randomised controlled trial. *Emergency Medicine Journal*, 35, 708–710.

Kudenchuk, P. J. et al. 2016. Amiodarone, lidocaine, or placebo in out-of-hospital cardiac arrest. *The New England Journal Of Medicine*, 374, 1711–1722.

Mann, C. J. 2003. Observational research methods. Research design II: Cohort, cross sectional, and case-control studies. *Emergency Medicine Journal*, 20, 54–60.

Moran, C. G. et al. 2018. Changing the system – Major trauma patients and their outcomes in the NHS (England) 2008–17. *Eclinicalmedicine*, 2–3, 13–21.

Nakahara, S. et al. 2013. Evaluation of prehospital administration of adrenaline (epinephrine) by emergency medical services for patients with out of hospital cardiac arrest in Japan: Controlled propensity matched retrospective cohort study. *BMJ*, 347, F6829.

National Institute for Health. n.d. NIH's definition of a clinical trial. Available at: https://grants.nih .gov/policy/clinical-trials/definition.htm [Accessed 28 April 2021].

National Institute for Health Research. 2019. Additional guidance for applicants including a clinical trial, pilot study or feasibility as part of a personal award application. Available at: https://www .nihr.ac.uk/documents/additional-guidance-for-applicants-including-a-clinical-trial-pilot-study -or-feasibility-as-part-of-a-personal-award-application/11702 [Accessed 29 April 2021].

Nichol, G. and Huszti, E. 2007. Design and implementation of resuscitation research: Special challenges and potential solutions. *Resuscitation*, 73, 337–346.

Nichol, G. et al. 2015. Trial of continuous or interrupted chest compressions during CPR. *The New England Journal of Medicine*, 373, 2203–2214.

Perkins, G. D. et al. 2015. Mechanical versus manual chest compression for out-of-hospital cardiac arrest (PARAMEDIC): A pragmatic, cluster randomised controlled trial. *Lancet*, 385, 947–955.

Perkins, G. D. et al. 2018. A randomized trial of epinephrine in out-of-hospital cardiac arrest. *The New England Journal of Medicine*, 379, 711–721.

Price, C. I. et al. 2020. Effect of an enhanced paramedic acute stroke treatment assessment on thrombolysis delivery during emergency stroke care: A cluster randomized clinical trial. *JAMA Neurology*, 77, 840–848.

Saquib, N., Saquib, J. and Ioannidis, J. P. 2013. Practices and impact of primary outcome adjustment in randomized controlled trials: Meta-epidemiologic study. *BMJ*, 347, F4313.

Schulz, K. F. et al. 2010. CONSORT 2010 statement: Updated guidelines for reporting parallel group randomised trials. *Trials*, 11, 32.

Schweizer, M. L., Braun, B. I. and Milstone, A. M. 2016. Research methods in healthcare epidemiology and antimicrobial stewardship-quasi-experimental designs. *Infection Control and Hospital Epidemiology*, 37, 1135–1140.

Sedgwick, P. 2014. Explanatory trials versus pragmatic trials. *BMJ*, 349, G6694.

Smith, I. M. et al. 2018. RePHILL: Protocol for a randomised controlled trial of prehospital blood product resuscitation for trauma. *Transfusion Medicine*, 28, 346–356.

Snooks, H. A. et al. 2017. Support and Assessment for Fall Emergency Referrals (SAFER) 2: A cluster randomised trial and systematic review of clinical effectiveness and cost-effectiveness of new protocols for emergency ambulance paramedics to assess older people following a fall with referral to community-based care when appropriate. *Health Technology Assessment*, 21, 1–218.

Stiell, I. G. et al. 2004. Advanced cardiac life support in out-of-hospital cardiac arrest. *The New England Journal of Medicine*, 351, 647–656.

Stiell, I. G. et al. 2011. Early versus later rhythm analysis in patients with out-of-hospital cardiac arrest. *The New England Journal Of Medicine*, 365, 787–797.

Torgerson, D. J. and Roberts, C. 1999. Understanding controlled trials. Randomisation methods: concealment. *BMJ*, 319, 375–376.

Chapter 6

Qualitative Research

Peter O'Meara and Dayne O'Meara

Chapter Objectives

The primary objective of this chapter is to enhance prehospital professionals' understanding and appreciation of qualitative research. Further reading and experience will be required to master specific qualitative research methods.

This chapter will cover:

- The value of qualitative research in the prehospital field
- The basic theoretical underpinnings of qualitative research
- An outline and examples of qualitative research methods used in the prehospital field
- Determining when to use qualitative methods
- An overview of the data collection and analytical tools used in qualitative research
- Frameworks designed to assess the trustworthiness of qualitative research

Introduction

When research is undertaken it is essential that both the design and the methods used are able to fully answer the research question under consideration (Kalu and Bwalya, 2017). The application of qualitative research is a long-standing and well-established research approach that uses non-numerical data to seek out and discover the perceived truths of phenomena across a wide spectrum of issues. It is a valuable approach when exploring complex phenomena that are difficult to measure quantitatively. Qualitative approaches are used in a range of disciplines to understand human experiences and situations, as well as individuals' cultures, beliefs and values; qualitative methods are used in anthropology and historical studies, contemporary cultural studies and more obviously in the political and marketing fields. Crucially, they are used to investigate many aspects of healthcare where the experiences, perspectives, beliefs and values of individuals or groups are important considerations.

Until relatively recently, prehospital researchers and the organisations that employ them eschewed qualitative research approaches in favour of more traditional

positivist approaches grounded in numerical data, seeking out the 'hard facts' (McLane and Chan, 2018). This reluctance to escape the safety of mainstream biomedical research methods to develop a stronger appreciation of the value of qualitative research methods in the prehospital domain is most probably related to the strong evidence-based clinical education and training that is dominant amongst emergency healthcare professionals. Without a broader research methods foundation in their curricula, it is difficult for clinical researchers and front-line health professionals to recognise and take full advantage of the strengths of qualitative research designs. In contrast to medicine, paramedicine and other emergency health professionals, general nursing has applied and valued qualitative research for longer and more consistently as a result of their very different foundational philosophies and values that place a high value on subjective patient and stakeholder experiences.

Apart from those found in nursing, many examples of prehospital qualitative research are found in graduate student-generated publications and dissertations. Its popularity and use continue to grow amongst mainstream prehospital researchers and health service researchers who are grappling with 'wicked problems' or issues that are highly resistant to resolution through traditional problem-solving approaches. One of the fundamental strengths of using qualitative approaches to answer research questions is their capacity to uncover silent issues and allow the voice of marginalised individuals and groups to be heard. They allow issues to be explored at a societal and cultural level within critical analysis frameworks that challenge the status quo.

For instance, Professor Julia Williams in the UK used qualitative techniques in her PhD to understand the relationship between homelessness and health status. Through reflexive interviews, she used individuals' narratives to identify their experiences of living on the streets. Linking together the findings of participants' lives and healthcare experiences were the constructs of inequality, disempowerment and marginalisation that contributed to social exclusion and homelessness (Williams, 2006). An Australian paramedic, Georgia Clarkson, employed a qualitative approach informed by a bricolage of critical theory (critique of society and culture) and hermeneutic **phenomenology** (which concerns the lived human experience), to explore the experiences of inclusion and marginalisation of gay and lesbian paramedics. Dr Clarkson found that participants were marginalised within their places of work and this had a detrimental impact on them, their colleagues, paramedic organisations and the communities they support (Clarkson, 2014).

The application of qualitative methods in these two studies illustrates how voices from the disadvantaged and marginalised can be recognised and heard using qualitative methods. Both these studies valued social context and listened to individual perspectives that were related to disadvantage. Their findings illuminated critical issues for health professionals and policy makers that would otherwise have been hidden from view.

When qualitative researchers conduct research and seek a version of the 'truth', they acknowledge the importance of their own experiences and observations of phenomena; in some cases, they draw conclusions from the absence of issues in the narratives as a result of limited information and knowledge, social taboos or more oppressive forms of social control. Qualitative researchers accept that difficult issues and new questions are likely to emerge from their engagement with participants and they therefore need to be diligently ethical and mindful of the harm they might inadvertently cause to participants and the communities they engage. Like other researchers, qualitative researchers' core ethical concerns are **informed consent**, confidentiality, anonymity and researchers' potential impact on the participants and vice versa (Goodwin et al., 2020; Sanjari et al., 2014).

There are potentially additional ethical concerns when qualitative research involves participant observation. Some have pointed out that while qualitative researchers do value informed consent, simply transferring the biomedical model of informed consent may be inappropriate to fully address the ethical concerns of some research designs (Bell, 2014; Fassin, 2006; Strathern, 2006). Rather than having participants sign a form at the beginning of their involvement as the main tool for gaining informed consent, consent may more primarily constitute an ongoing conversation that evolves based on major events occurring in a community during fieldwork (O'Meara, 2020). If a research design is chosen that blurs the lines between research and personal relationships, then the researcher may have other ethical obligations to participants beyond the confines of research activities (High, 2011).

Unlike quantitative researchers, qualitative researchers do not propose a hypothesis to prove or disprove. Instead, they bring a premise for their research based on the available evidence and their own values and experiences. These underlying principles are why field trips (observation), building trust (empathetic listening) and immersion in communities (gaining perspective) are important components of qualitative research design, implementation and reporting. In some instances, there are important cultural and organisational barriers to consider which obscure participants' perception and understanding of worlds other than the one they live and work in.

A prehospital example of a constraining factor has been observed in the USA where paramedics and Emergency Medical Services (EMS) medical directors are deeply invested in the 'medical direction' model for EMS (National Association of EMS Physicians and National Association of State EMS Officials, 2010). Both physicians and paramedics consider that this model of oversight is an essential element of effective and safe EMS systems. In contrast, paramedic systems in the UK and Australia operate effectively and safely under the banner of clinical governance where medical dominance is moderated through paramedic leadership (O'Meara et al., 2017; O'Meara et al., 2018).

Theoretical Underpinnings

Qualitative researchers are arguably more concerned with the formation and application of theoretical frameworks than quantitative researchers. These frameworks help qualitative researchers and their readers to better understand their findings, discussion and conclusions. Having a theoretical position prior to undertaking the research helps structure the research process; while debated, it is generally accepted that theory in qualitative research acts as an initial guide to research design, data collection processes and techniques, as well as informing researchers about how data will be analysed and interpreted (Kalu and Bwalya, 2017). A researcher's theoretical stance is the product of their worldview, in particular their position about the nature of society, knowledge and understanding. Their **epistemological** stance inevitably influences all stages of the research process. In a well-designed qualitative research study, **bias** of this type can be avoided or mitigated through researchers clearly identifying their own epistemological stance (Kalu and Bwalya, 2017).

This focus on theoretical underpinnings can be off-putting to many in the prehospital field, where their efforts tend to be concentrated on facilitating access to evidence-based interventions and appropriate follow-up care. It is rare for prehospital leaders and clinicians to see or discuss theoretical models; as a result, few prehospital models have been developed or widely discussed.

One example of a theoretical model that has been developed and shared through the literature is Campeau's Space Control Theory for paramedicine that uses context to analyse and explain how paramedics work in a unique setting that requires a unique set of knowledge and skills (Campeau, 2008a, 2008b, 2009). This study used a **grounded theory** methodology to conduct a qualitative inquiry that involved interviewing paramedics across different levels of experience about their approach to scene management. The result was the development of a formal theory of paramedic scene management.

A growing proportion of the qualitative research in the prehospital field is now coming from paramedics who have completed or are currently undertaking doctoral studies examining the meaning of their emerging profession and how they interact with culturally diverse populations, transforming workforces and complex health systems. In Australia, where entry-to-practice Baccalaureate degree and graduate research programmes are well-established, a growing group of paramedic researchers have extensively used qualitative methods to build the theoretical foundations of the paramedic profession (Reynolds, 2008; Clarkson, 2014; Devenish, 2014; Furness, 2018; Hartley, 2012; O'Meara et al., 2012a; Long, 2017).

Louise Reynolds, in a seminal study, used ethnographic techniques to better understand and communicate organisational cultural issues within a State-wide ambulance service (Reynolds, 2008, 2009). Dr Reynolds used grand and constituent metaphors for an organisational culture while addressing the paucity of research relating to the ambulance industry in Australia at that time. Thematic analysis of the transcripts was used to develop a conceptual framework that enabled a description of this culture. A feature and strength of the research was the insider perspective of taken-for-granted assumptions and practices that are part of working 'in ambulance'.

'The thesis contributes to the body of knowledge in the health care and management disciplines that also "goes beyond" the notion that ambulance workers are merely "stretcher bearers" or "drivers" for the medical profession and the community, and acknowledges that their contribution is important to the health outcomes of community members'

(Reynolds, 2008).

In the UK, Andy Newton used mixed methods to consider the future of paramedics following their professionalisation and registration as health professionals. Dr Newton initially surveyed paramedics to determine how they rated their training and to establish their attitudes to a more educationally based approach. Following environmental changes in the health system, strategic foresight and horizon scanning were employed to detect 'signals', themes and trends in relation to newly emerging 'competitors' to the paramedic role. This approach allowed consideration of factors such as professional power in an environment where there was a reluctance to acknowledge the emerging issues and the limited evidence base (Newton, 2014). This work has resulted in discussions and debates that have challenged the paramedic profession and the wider prehospital field to imagine alternative futures (Newton and Harris, 2015; Newton, 2012; Newton, 2011).

Nursing and allied health researchers have employed qualitative research methods in the prehospital field. Australian physiotherapist Dr Sophie Anaf used observational data to understand the shift in professional physiotherapy roles in emergency department settings. She used an intensive five-day observational, single-case design that collected researcher observations and the features of patient interventions provided by physiotherapists (Anaf and Sheppard, 2007). The same research team undertook a review of the qualitative literature to better understand the patient experience in the emergency department that highlighted caring or the lack of caring in regard to the patients' psychological and emotional needs, rather than the common concerns about emergency department 'medical-technical' skill and efficiency (Gordon et al., 2010).

There are numerous accounts of the utilisation of qualitative methods in nursing related to prehospital settings. One example with contemporary relevance to prehospital health professionals is an Irish study that was undertaken to determine nurses' perceptions of the factors that cause violence and aggression in the emergency department. In this study, 12 emergency department nurses were interviewed. Thematic analysis of the interview data identified that environmental and communication factors contributed to aggression, and that triage was the area in the emergency department where aggression was most likely to occur (Angland et al., 2014). From this study, a number of useful recommendations were made to improve the safety of emergency department staff.

Qualitative Research Designs

It is common for qualitative research in prehospital settings to employ generic qualitative approaches, such as thematic analysis, for pragmatic reasons, with the attendant risk that studies might lack high levels of rigour (Cooper and Endacott,

2007). For this reason, it is necessary to continue developing qualitative research skills in the prehospital field and to strive for qualitative research 'best practice'. The growing success of qualitative studies in emergency healthcare settings has resulted in specific recommendations for how to undertake qualitative research in the prehospital and emergency settings, with the most commonly recommended research designs being **ethnography, grounded theory** and **phenomenology** (Cooper et al., 2009). In addition, prehospital researchers successfully employ historical research techniques, **action research** methodologies and mixed methods that often incorporate case study design characteristics.

The choice of qualitative research design is dependent upon the purpose of the study and the specific research questions, as well as an understanding of the setting and context. The research design needs to be described in simple language and to include the rationale for the qualitative approach adopted, how data will be gathered and analysed, as well as any ethical or pragmatic considerations that have influenced the design. The settings in which studies are conducted matters; prehospital settings have their own set of characteristics, including limited time and urgency to act, that need to be considered when choosing research approaches (Cooper et al., 2009).

Ethnography

The goal of ethnographic research is to understand people's cultures, beliefs and values through immersion of the researcher in a given community or environment, ideally over an extended period of time (**Box 6.1**). A robust ethnography written as a book or thesis is traditionally based on one to two years of continuous fieldwork, although shorter periods of research may still be conducted ethnographically. There is no single procedure to follow when using ethnography; however, it is a field-oriented activity that has cultural interpretations at its core (Lambert et al., 2011). This approach has historically been characteristic of the discipline of anthropology, but it has also become a popular research methodology in other social sciences and humanities. Early ethnographies often took place in colonial settings, with the long-term nature of ethnographic research made necessary to enable the researcher

---

Box 6.1 Ethnographers and Ethnographic Designs

An ethnographer is a researcher who makes use of an ethnographic research design. The word ethnography may be used to refer to the associated suite of research methods – *doing* or *using* ethnography – or it may be used to refer to the research output of a project using ethnographic methods. The specific combination of methods used in an ethnographic project must be determined by the researcher depending on the research setting and the researcher's own capabilities. An ethnographic project will usually involve some combination of interviews, focus groups, surveys, photography, film, case studies and participant observation.

to learn local languages from scratch and to come to grips with entire social worlds that were vastly different to their own in almost every regard (Evans-Pritchard, 1937; Malinowski, 1922). Since its beginnings in British colonial anthropology, ethnography has come to be valued in a wide range of field sites, both within anthropology and beyond. It has been successfully used to study businesses, global religions, educational institutions, places of work, small-scale social structures, vast urban landscapes and more.

Ethnography is valued due to its effectiveness at accessing an extraordinary *depth* of information from research participants – this may be valuable on its own, or it may complement other forms of data collection that offer a greater *breadth* of information, such as through quantitative methods or surveys of larger populations. For populations and topics that are logistically difficult to engage solely using interviews or other more structured methods, ethnography may present the most practical way to gain access to a particular worldview. It is also effective for studying cultural dynamics that a population may not be aware of or may not entirely understand themselves; a research participant may not be able to fully articulate complex ongoing cultural dynamics that they take for granted, but an ethnographer may observe connections between events or ideas in practice.

Arguably the most important method of data collection pioneered by ethnographers is participant observation. Participant observation means that the researcher will spend extended periods of time immersed in the research setting, recognised and accepted by informants as a social actor who has some part to play in ongoing professional, social or economic activities while simultaneously conducting research. For ethnographers studying the culture of a remote village, this may mean that they assist with ongoing agricultural or ritual activities that are relevant to the research questions being investigated. They may be placed into local kinship networks and be expected to act accordingly. Ethnography in a medical or healthcare field may utilise participant observation by having the researcher accompany paramedics on callouts, assist with administrative work at a hospital or take part in conversations between patients, doctors and nurses. Listening to patients' and staff members' own ideas of their situation, medical condition, feelings and perceptions – especially while embedded in that context – provides the researcher with the means to uncover emic perspectives on the research topic and then integrate that with their own etic perspective (**Box 6.2**).

Ethnography has been described as an exercise in 'thick description' (Geertz, 1973). This means not resting at simply capturing what took place or what was said. Ethnographers must work to uncover the spoken and unspoken meanings attached to cultural beliefs and practices documented in the field. This is a process that cannot take place in later stages of analysis. If field notes or interview transcripts are missing key aspects of sociocultural context as embedded in that moment in space and time, then the analysis may misconstrue what took place by neglecting emic interpretations. Interpretive thick description must therefore begin while in the field. An ethnographer's embodied memory of field experiences and background contextual knowledge will inevitably play a role in analysis, but thorough

Box 6.2 Emic Versus Etic Language Rules

The terms emic and etic originate in linguistics, taken from the words phonemic and phonetic, respectively (Pike, 1967); emic language rules are those articulated and consciously adhered to by native speakers, while etic language rules are those that can be triangulated by an observing linguist but may be of little relevance to the speakers themselves (Markee, 2013). These terms have since been used extensively by anthropologists to describe the different perspectives on cultural systems that come to light through ethnographic research (Harris, 1976). Emic and etic are sometimes glossed as 'insider' and 'outsider' perspectives, respectively. Participant observation is designed to integrate these two perspectives in data collection and analysis.

ethnographic notetaking in the field will result in raw data that include the thick descriptions necessary to assist in fuller analyses at a later date. This aspect of ethnographic research leads to the dual meaning of ethnography as referring to both method and published text; the analysis and production of text begins to take form at the time of data collection and then continues when the ethnographer leaves the field. The ultimate goal of this interpretive approach is to reveal the logic underlying particular actions, events and ideas by interpreting what is observed, what informants have to say, how this relates to prior observations, as well as what ethnographers themselves experience through their own participation in the field.

An important part of the interpretive process in ethnography is recognising the role played by the researcher's own subjectivity in their engagement with social actors in the field. Ethnographers themselves become deeply involved in the nature of data collected in a much more nuanced way than if they were simply the person conducting an interview. As ethnographic research is designed to be inherently interpretive, this kind of subjectivity is not something to be eliminated as in other methodologies more common in biomedical fields, but, rather, something to be acknowledged at the outset and factored into the analysis accordingly. This means that two ethnographers doing research in the same field site may come up with very different insights or pursue very different topics. This is a normal feature of ethnography and is not problematic so long as the ethnographer's interpretive process and theoretical framework are made clear in the final research output. Because participant observation requires the researcher to involve themselves in the cultural processes under study, the researcher's personal background may have profound effects on the nature of the study. If a researcher holds considerable privilege compared to a marginalised community they are studying, then they may need to reflect on the difference in their experience of the field site compared to that of their informants (Duneier, 2000). The way that informants perceive the researcher and thereby situate them in existing webs of social relationships can both influence the direction of a project and be enlightening regarding the ways that people there make sense of the world around them (Bornstein, 2007; Venkatesh, 2002).

In medical fields, nursing in particular has embraced ethnography as a research methodology to explore the nature of the profession and to better understand patient experiences (Lambert et al., 2011). A Finnish study used ethnography to identify and explore the actions, experiences and perceptions of community nurse-paramedics (CNPs) within their sphere of practice (Rasku et al., 2020). The context of this study was a newly implemented government programme that saw professionals in emergency and prehospital nursing transition into newly created one-person community paramedicine units. Researchers aimed to improve understanding of this particular healthcare model. They used inductive content analysis to identify key themes that emerged from the interview and participant observation data. The study concluded that CNPs need the right attitude to engage in the more prolonged care relationship with patients compared to prior roles in the emergency medical response. CNPs also benefited from additional skills training to improve their ability to assist palliative care patients whom they did not have extensive prior experience with. This allowed CNPs to offer a valuable preventative care service that was greatly appreciated by patients' families. The authors identified two main reasons for choosing an ethnographic research design: ethnography's ability to generate deep understanding of highly situated topics, and its effectiveness at studying cultural change. It was important to the researchers that they be able to record not only quantitatively measurable **outcomes** of this policy, but also the community and worker sentiments towards its implementation.

Grounded Theory

Grounded theory is an inductive research design that originated in the discipline of sociology. 'Grounded theory' is not actually a single theory, but, rather, a method for collecting and analysing data in order to build theory. It makes use of qualitative data, which are analysed and then used to develop theories that are grounded in the data (Kalu and Bwalya, 2017). Carefully transcribed interviews are a key component of grounded theory, allowing for the data to be systematically coded by the researcher for a comprehensive process of content analysis. Observation often plays a key role as well. Recurrent themes in interviews and observed interactions are identified and used to inform the development of a 'grounded theory' that is emergent from the data rather than based on theoretical frameworks developed in other contexts (Charmaz, 2014). This ensures that the 'fit' of the theory will be appropriate, being able to explain phenomena rather than being forced onto phenomena as an explanation (Urquhart, 2019). Much like with ethnography, the analytical process of grounded theory begins in fieldwork and depends upon the researcher being present in a particular social setting where events are unfolding in practice.

Grounded theory was first used in a sociological study led by Barney Glaser and Anselm Strauss: *Awareness of Dying* (Glaser and Strauss, 1966). The aim of their study was to learn about how people interact with one another when someone is dying, particularly how doctors and nurses in the USA communicate or fail to communicate with patients and their families on the subject of impending death and how dying is 'managed' as an institutional process in healthcare. Glaser and

Strauss pursued this topic based on their observation that death was a topic often consciously avoided in US hospitals at the time. They suspected there would be particular interactional dynamics depending on who knew what about a patient's impending death, and this was borne out by the results of their study. Since the 1960s, there has been a shift to 'open awareness' of death as the standard practice in US hospitals, but there are particular areas of medicine and healthcare where it remains an avoided topic, giving continued relevance to the grounded theory developed in the earlier context (Stacey et al., 2019).

The methodology developed by Glaser and Strauss was described in more detail in a separate book, *The Discovery of Grounded Theory*, published two years after their original study (Glaser and Strauss, 1967). They noted that much sociological work in the past had been preoccupied with generating theories and then working to verify their accuracy. What Glaser and Strauss described as a grounded theory would make the step of verification unnecessary, as any theory in such a study would come directly from the data. The pursuit of grounded theory was proposed as an exercise in comparative analysis, as opposed to experimental or statistical methods. Glaser and Strauss emphasised that their approach to comparative analysis would not restrict the units for comparison to large-scale social units as was customary in both sociology and anthropology at the time. They saw value in engaging in comparative analysis on a smaller scale, such as for wards in a hospital or classes in a school (Glaser and Strauss, 1967).

Grounded theory, like ethnography, is an inductive research design in which the process of analysis begins during fieldwork. Both grounded theory and ethnography are effective at revealing insights about the emic perspective of the issue under investigation (Aldiabat and Navenec, 2011). However, where ethnography is typically interested in understanding a particular group of people, grounded theory is more focused on understanding a particular type of interaction. Grounded theory depends on highly systematic coding of data and typically involves less participation in the field site. Observation is an important form of data collection alongside other methods but, compared to ethnography, the researcher takes a less active role in the production of data (Timmermans and Tavory, 2007). The researcher's own interpretations of events in the field are therefore afforded less importance in grounded theory research designs. Much of the data that ethnographers collect through participant observation may include things less conducive to text-based coding, such as remembered informal conversations that were unable to be accurately recorded, emotional experiences of the ethnographer or visual cues from people or objects that are imbued with meaning. While anthropologists using ethnography often adhere to the maxim that 'everything is data', sociologists using grounded theory have a set of processes that clearly delineate what is and is not data for the purposes of analysis (**Box 6.3**).

Given grounded theory's origins in hospital research and its focus on interactions between people not necessarily of the same cultural group, it is a research design that is popular in qualitative research relating to healthcare. David Long, an Australian

Box 6.3 Grounded Theory Coding and Analysis

Just as the theory emerges from the data in grounded theory research, so too do the codes used at the beginning stages of analysis. Material collected at the beginning of fieldwork is analysed by the researcher to identify the first codes that will be used with subsequently collected material. This process continues throughout fieldwork. A code may be a particular theme that research participants consistently raise, or key words and phrases that come up frequently in interview transcripts. This allows the researcher to classify these selections of the material as salient data and then group together similar data in later stages of analysis. This differs from some other qualitative research designs where the codes applied to interview transcripts may have been deductively anticipated by the researcher before data collection based on prior studies or particular research questions (Flick, 2018). Grounded theory is also characterised by 'memos' written by the researcher. In grounded theory research, a memo refers to a highly focused type of field note that is compiled in order to document the ongoing process of coded category creation in conjunction with the collection of data (Flick, 2018).

paramedic, used a grounded theory methodology to illuminate how qualified paramedics transitioned to a specialist role in community paramedicine in Australia and Canada (Long, 2017). In community paramedicine, the underlying philosophy is the provision of more healthcare options to patients in the community so that they can readily navigate the health system and, where possible, avoid emergency department visits. The challenge in this study was the lack of knowledge and understanding of the paramedic transition from traditional emergency response roles to that of a specialist community paramedic. This study built on the work of other researchers in nursing and paramedicine who had previously considered work-role transition theories. Its strength was the stronger focus on the complex interplay between the elements, core categories and phases that comprise the community paramedicine transition experience. This was achieved through the systematic method offered by grounded theory to understand interactional dynamics. Through these efforts, Dr Long's study made a significant contribution to the understanding of how paramedics transition to community paramedicine and generated targeted intervention points for paramedics to navigate the transition experience more efficiently.

Phenomenology

Phenomenology is a research design that is rooted in philosophy and commonly used in a range of social and health sciences (**Box 6.4**). Phenomenological research typically relies heavily on interviews but often incorporates observational methods of data collection as well. The purpose of phenomenology is to understand the common meaning attached to a particular phenomenon by research participants who have experienced it. It was originally proposed as a 'rigorous descriptive

Box 6.4 Phenomenological Research

Phenomenology is focused on understanding what is referred to as people's 'lived experiences'. This means interrogating people's recollections of what it was like living through a particular phenomenon. The phenomenon under investigation will be something that is universally experienced within the population under study. Phenomenological research reveals the common essence of how research participants come to attach meaning to phenomena.

science of consciousness' (Baker et al., 1992). This pursuit of description rather than explanation or analysis is driven by an underlying epistemological assumption that rejects Cartesian dualism of subject–object distinctions. A key premise of phenomenological research is that due to the subjective nature of human experience, the reality of phenomena is only accessible through the subjective consciousness of those who experience it (Creswell and Poth, 2016). Phenomenology is thus based more on revealing subjective meaning than developing abstract theories (Flood, 2010).

Phenomenology can be broadly divided into either descriptive or interpretive phenomenology. Descriptive phenomenology is the older approach, based directly on the philosophy of Husserl, who is credited as the founder of phenomenology (Husserl, 1970; Wojnar and Swanson, 2007). In descriptive phenomenology, the researcher strives to remove any personal bias based on their own prior experiences and to capture a pure and universal description of the phenomenon that is aligned with the lived experiences of participants. The process of setting aside the researcher's subjectivity is known as bracketing. This will, theoretically, lead the researcher to uncover universal essences of understanding that phenomenon. Interpretive phenomenology, also called hermeneutic phenomenology, was developed by Husserl's successors and is particularly credited to Heidegger, one of his students (Wojnar and Swanson, 2007; Heidegger, 1962). Heidegger's interpretive phenomenology placed a greater emphasis on situating lived experiences in the appropriate context, aiming to provide greater rigour to phenomenological research. The role of culture, social context and historical period as being either peripheral or central to understanding phenomena is the key difference between descriptive and interpretive phenomenology.

When compared with grounded theory and ethnography, there are again some key distinctions to be aware of when choosing which research design or combination of research designs is most suitable for a particular qualitative research study. Ethnographers have found benefits to phenomenological approaches that shift the researcher's focus away from the collective systems and social structures of a cultural group to explorations of individual consciousness that may be otherwise neglected (Baker et al., 1992; Eberle, 2015; Katz and Csordas, 2003). Grounded theory is also conventionally better suited to social structures, with phenomenology designed for research that is more interested in psychological structures. Grounded theory and phenomenology often take a similar approach to eliminating or minimising researcher subjectivity through bracketing practices, but the underlying reasoning for doing so is quite different. Phenomenology's goal is to reveal the essential meaning of a phenomenon, and this requires the researcher to set themselves aside. In grounded theory, the researcher brackets their own preconceptions and predispositions in order to remove extraneous factors that could affect the utility of explanatory theory that is built from the data (Starks and Brown Trinidad, 2007).

Phenomenological methodologies can be successfully applied to clinical questions. One example comes from the UK, where a research team used a constructivist view and an interpretive phenomenological approach to better understand the treatment of pain (Iqbal et al., 2013). The research team conducted interviews and focus groups of patients, paramedics and emergency department clinicians to ascertain the lived experiences of those involved in the prehospital management of pain. Participants were asked to describe their experiences during these healthcare episodes and to explain what it meant to them and how the identified facilitators and/or barriers associated with the management of pain might be improved. The researchers found that there was much uncertainty surrounding the experience of prehospital pain due to communication difficulties between patients, paramedics and hospital clinicians, and the difficulty of accurately measuring the intensity of pain. For paramedics, assessing pain and deciding how to proceed involved carefully weighing multiple sources of information. Patients often felt confused or uninformed about the questions asked of them and the pain alleviation options available. The researchers, by improving their understanding of prehospital pain management, were able to make a number of specific recommendations to improve patient and paramedic experiences of this phenomenon.

Phenomenology was particularly well suited to this study because the subject of research – pain – is a phenomenon that is inherently subjective and therefore hard to measure in a universal way. The researchers sought to reveal key essences of this subjective phenomenon that would be applicable to the context of prehospital care in the UK. Other research designs were not chosen in this case because the researchers were not seeking to analyse causes of the issue or to build theory to explain some aspect of it. They measured people's perception of the phenomenon and learned what those people's preferences were regarding it moving forward. In cases where there is a discrete subjective phenomenon like this, phenomenology offers an effective toolkit for problem solving in clinical practice.

Other Common Qualitative Approaches to Research

Apart from the previously discussed qualitative approaches, including related methodologies, prehospital qualitative researchers employ a wide range of strategies to answer their research questions and make improvements to systems and processes. They employ, either separately or in combination: the techniques of historians and journalists to learn from the past; action research to help design, implement and evaluate system innovations; and mixed methods and case studies to better understand phenomena.

Historical research techniques can help build a body of professional knowledge and better understand professional roles, along with enhancing our understanding of the economic, legal and political context that has constructed the accepted truth. This approach involves systematic collection, evaluation and synthesising of historic data to understand past events and then relate it to contemporary circumstances and visions of the future. The product of this historical research is often seen in the introductory statements of research **proposals** and papers that help locate the research context (Llewellyn, 2017). For example, an Australian paramedic, Scott Devenish, searched archival documents to explore the heroic role of Australian stretcher bearers during the First World War as a reflection on the evolution of the modern paramedic (Devenish and O'Meara, 2010).

Action research is an approach commonly used for improving conditions and practices in healthcare environments (Lingard et al., 2008; Whitehead et al., 2003). It involves healthcare practitioners conducting systematic enquiries in order to help them improve their own practices, which in turn can enhance their working environment and the working environments of clients, patients and users. Its strength lies in its focus on generating solutions to practical problems and its ability to empower practitioners, by getting them to engage with research and the subsequent development of implementation activities. The collection and synthesis of qualitative data is an important component of most action research projects as a consequence of its participatory characteristics. This methodology has been used in the UK to improve emergency care pathways (Endacott et al., 2011). In this study, the research team combined retrospective patient data, interviews with staff, observation of patient pathways and measurement of team climate that exposed gaps and inconsistencies in emergency department working practices.

Just as action research was used as part of a mixed methods project in the emergency department example above, it can be used in combination with case study techniques. In Australia, a research team exploring the emergence of new paramedic practice roles has used action research to capture the complex and interconnected place of paramedics in rural communities. Following thematic analysis that used the sociological framework as a filter, the study found that paramedics are increasingly becoming first-line primary healthcare providers in small rural communities and developing additional professional responsibilities throughout the cycle of care (O'Meara et al., 2012b).

Mixed methods in prehospital research are relatively new, although **case study research** is relatively common and shares some of the same characteristics. Case study research is a qualitative approach in which the researcher explores a bounded system or systems over time. In-depth data is collected from multiple sources such as observations, interviews, audio-visual material, documents and reports. Each case is described and often presented after thematic analysis.

According to researchers in the field, the prehospital field is embracing mixed methods as an approach to research because of its ability to address healthcare questions in complex, diverse environments (McManamny et al., 2015). The qualitative component of **mixed methods research** is a useful tool that can help interpret quantitative study findings or generate further research questions by identifying participants' motivations and feelings (Ingham et al., 2014). Qualitative methods are often applied to data collected through open-question surveys to add to quantitative data. For instance, paramedic researcher Brian Maguire has used thematic and content analysis techniques to explore potential strategies to reduce violence in the prehospital workplace and then placed the finding into a theoretical framework that was shared to form an evidence base for prevention of workplace violence (Maguire et al., 2018).

The Mechanics of Qualitative Research

Qualitative researchers need to systematically demonstrate transparency and accountability throughout the whole research process so that users of research findings are able to clearly see the decision-making and the analytical approach (Kalu and Bwalya, 2017). As is the case with quantitative research, having a well-thought-out research plan that maps the research process from beginning to end is a good way to achieve this aim. Qualitative researchers need to demonstrate transparency and accountability throughout the process of (Kalu and Bwalya, 2017):

- Choosing the research topic
- Defining the research question
- Justifying the research appropriateness
- Stating the adoption of the theory
- Outlining the research design
- Choosing the sample and sampling strategy
- Methods of data collection
- Analysis of data
- Applying consideration to research ethics
- Demonstrating data trustworthiness
- Reflexivity.

Fully understanding all of these qualitative research elements is beyond the scope of this relatively short chapter. The following sections describe two important components of qualitative research methods that need to be understood, namely data collection and analysis of data.

Data Collection

Whether researchers are using ethnography (including auto-ethnography), grounded theory, phenomenology or other approaches to qualitative research, they have a wide range of data collection techniques available to them. Prehospital qualitative researchers collect data through observations during field visits (including video recordings), individual and group interviews, focus groups or self-reflection through storytelling. In addition, qualitative researchers often examine historical or policy documents to find answers to their research questions, while another common means of collecting qualitative data is through open-ended survey questions that are often combined with closed questions (mixed methods).

Using creative variations of these data collection approaches can be seen in the prehospital research when questions are hard to openly discuss, debate or answer. For instance, an Australian prehospital research team creatively adapted and combined focus groups and community conversation approaches drawn from the Nelson Mandela Foundation (Nelson Mandela Foundation (NMF), 2009) and the Indigenous Leadership Network in Victoria (Stone-Resneck, 2010), amongst others, to examine the duration and variation in quality of paramedic student placements over several days (Hickson et al., 2014; O'Meara et al., 2014). Community conversations are structured, inclusive conversations rather than consultations that bring together a group of people to engage in meaningful conversation, share knowledge and ideas and discuss potential solutions to complex problems. The participants in this study included paramedics, ambulance service managers, paramedicine students and paramedicine educators who were attending a conference on paramedic education and leadership. The conversations took place over three days, with participants spending around five hours discussing the key issues related to paramedicine student clinical placements. Participants were formed into small groups and then invited to discuss the quality in paramedicine student clinical placements and asked to propose possible solutions. The research aim was to engage all the stakeholders in meaningful conversations that promoted and shared knowledge and ideas to generate innovative solutions.

This series of conversations about clinical education was fluid and flexible and the processes evolved continuously and dynamically, letting ideas emerge in a way that resulted in the conversation continuing once participants had left the conference. Feedback from participants was positive and supported the concept of community conversations; they enjoyed meaningful conversations, shared their collective intelligence and engaged more deeply with the critical issues. Participants considered the community conversation approach as a valuable learning tool that led to creative and innovative solutions. In addition, the conversations were seen as a way for participants to be more actively involved than is usual at conferences when passive, lecture-style approaches are the norm (Hickson et al., 2014).

Analysis of Data

There are many approaches used to analyse qualitative data; arguably the most often used and understood in the prehospital field is thematic analysis. It aims to develop a description of the patterns of response in a dataset that capture important information about the research question (Braun and Clarke, 2006). Thematic analysis is a foundational method for qualitative analysis and provides core skills that are shared across a broad range of qualitative methods. It is generally considered the first qualitative method of analysis that researchers should learn, as it provides core skills that will be useful for conducting other forms of qualitative analysis (Holloway and Todres, 2003).

The advantages of thematic analysis include its flexibility and the relative ease with which those with limited qualitative research experience are able to learn in a short timeframe with the help of experienced mentors. Because thematic analysis can summarise key features of a large body of data and offer rich descriptions, research findings are more accessible to the general public. Another advantage is that it can be used within the participatory **research paradigm** where participants, whether they are health professionals or patients, work as collaborators or co-designers. As a result of these and other strengths, thematic analysis is well suited to informing policy development (Braun and Clarke, 2006).

Qualitative analytic methods can be roughly divided into two philosophical camps: inductive, where codes and themes are based on the data collected; and deductive, where an existing framework is used to categorise and make sense of data. Both have strengths and weaknesses that need to be considered during the design stage of projects.

An inductive approach is data driven, with themes identified that are strongly linked to the data themselves and not necessarily bearing a strong relationship to the specific questions that were asked of the participants. Uncovering surprises is an attractive feature of the inductive analytic process, with the findings not being driven by the researchers' theoretical interest in the area or topic, or a pre-existing position or framework. However, it is important to acknowledge that researchers cannot completely free themselves of their theoretical and epistemological commitments. In contrast, a deductive approach to thematic analysis tends to be driven by the researcher's theoretical or analytic interest in the area and is thus more explicitly researcher driven. This form of thematic analysis tends to provide a less rich description of the data overall, and more a detailed analysis of some aspect of the data (Braun and Clarke, 2006). Irrespective of which approach is taken to thematic analysis, it is important to recognise that researchers tend to and should become immersed in the data, generating initial codes, searching for themes, reviewing themes, defining and naming themes and producing a written report. There are several well-known software programmes available to support this synthesis process that require specialised training.

Paramedic Peter Hartley used a combination of narrative enquiry and thematic analysis to investigate the purpose, nature and satisfaction of paramedic practices as they related to an awareness of the cultural and religious needs of diverse community groups (Hartley, 2012). Through structured interviews and a focus group, Dr Hartley collected data that incorporated the voices of community groups on their experiences with emergency paramedics during prehospital healthcare in Melbourne,

Australia. Two independent volunteer groups participated: community groups incorporating representatives from the African, Asian, Middle Eastern, Muslim, Jewish and Indigenous Australian communities; and paramedic practitioners. Using inductive analysis, Hartley identified themes that indicated that the paramedics had both a deficit of knowledge and a presence of incorrect knowledge about cultural practices that impacted directly on their professional practice. The paramedic participants recognised many of these shortfalls and identified that there was a lack of useful cross-cultural education and training available to them. The study recommended strategies to improve interventions with diverse community groups in the prehospital setting and identified areas of cross-cultural curricula that should be incorporated into paramedic education.

Choosing a Qualitative Research Approach

Prehospital practitioners or researchers without specific training or experience in qualitative research methods face the dilemma of how to determine the qualitative approach that is best suited to their research question. Do they choose grounded theory, ethnography, phenomenology or some other approach that employs related qualitative methods? Arguably, the most important step is to initially consider how their view of the world or epistemological stance will affect their approach. Alignment between the researchers' worldviews, the belief system underpinning the research approach and the research question is a prerequisite for rigorous and worthwhile qualitative research.

In the short term, prehospital researchers with limited qualitative research backgrounds can take the following steps to inform their decisions: firstly, examine the existing literature and note what is known about the topic and which approaches have previously been used; secondly, find a qualitatively skilled collaborator and talk to them about the needs of the project as well as some background about the prehospital field; thirdly, following completion of the first two steps, decide which qualitative approach is best suited to answering the research question. Questions to consider during this decision-making process include (Teherani et al., 2015):

- Will the findings contribute to the creation of a theoretical model to better understand the area of study? (grounded theory)

- Will the researcher(s) need to spend an extended amount of time trying to understand the culture and processes of prehospital systems? (ethnography)

- Is there a particular phenomenon that needs to be better understood or described? (phenomenology)

In the longer term, prehospital researchers could invest in continuing education. This can be through obtaining and reading a qualitative research textbook or undertaking an online course. However, probably the most valuable approach is to collaborate with a qualitative researcher who can provide mentorship and support. Once the basics of qualitative research are learnt, a good way of experientially consolidating knowledge and skills is to undertake a small-scale pilot study with the support of a qualitative expert (Teherani et al., 2015). This will provide an appreciation of the thought processes that contribute to study design, data analysis and reporting the findings. This experience might lead to other opportunities to become a team member of a larger study led by a qualitative expert.

What is Good Qualitative Research?

While some argue that qualitative research can and should be assessed with reference to the same broad criteria of quality as quantitative research, others argue that qualitative research should be judged against its own standards and characteristics. This is an important debate in the health sector where questions of 'rigour' are highly valued in the context of '**evidence-based practice**'. The issue of 'quality' in qualitative research is part of a much larger and contested debate about the nature of the knowledge produced by qualitative research, whether its quality can legitimately be judged according to a single framework or set of general principles.

It is agreed that for qualitative research to be judged as good research, there is a need for transparency, accountability and reflexivity on the part of researchers to explicitly account for all decisions made throughout the research process. This starts from determining the research topic and goes through to the conclusions reached. Researchers need to exhibit clarity and responsibility, as well as reflecting on their influence as a researcher on the research process. All good qualitative research must inform the readers of decisions made at all stages of the research process (Kalu and Bwalya, 2017). As a result of these questions, there has been a proliferation of guidelines for undertaking and judging qualitative research in the same way that quantitative research is evaluated and reported. For example, a 32-item checklist (the COnsolidated criteria for REporting Qualitative research (COREQ)) for interviews and focus groups has been developed and validated to report qualitative research (Tong et al., 2007). Further to this, the ENTREQ (enhancing transparency in reporting the synthesis of qualitative research) statement has been developed to help researchers report the stages commonly associated with the synthesis of qualitative health research (Tong et al., 2012).

In Australia, emergency medicine researchers have made a methodological contribution to the ongoing debate about rigour in qualitative research methods studies through the application of what they describe as the four-dimensional criteria to assess the rigour of their mixed methods research project examining the implementation of a government policy on an emergency department time target (Forero et al., 2018). They assessed the robustness of their study on the basis of credibility, dependability, confirmability and transferability, which have previously been described and are widely used amongst qualitative researchers. These criteria for determining the trustworthiness of qualitative research were introduced in the 1980s to replace rigour, **reliability**, validity and **generalisability** – criteria that are more associated with quantitative research.

More recently, this four-dimensional criteria approach has been critiqued, with recommendations to return to the traditional criteria with the suggestion that specific strategies can be used to achieve high levels of rigour. The suggested good practice strategies are: prolonged engagement, persistent observation and thick, rich description; **inter-rater reliability**, negative case analysis; peer review or debriefing; clarifying researcher bias; member checking; external audits; and **triangulation** (Morse, 2015). The debate around reporting criteria is likely to be ongoing, given the inherent difficulty associated with the undefined and fluctuating nature of qualitative research.

> 'Qualitative research is expansive and occasionally controversial, spanning many different methods of inquiry and epistemological approaches. A "one-size-fits-all" standard for reporting qualitative research can be restrictive, but COREQ and SRQR [Standards for Reporting Qualitative Research] both serve as valuable tools for developing responsible qualitative research proposals, effectively communicating research decisions, and evaluating submissions. Ultimately, tailoring a set of standards specific to health design research and its frequently used methods would ensure quality research and aid reviewers in their evaluations'

> (Peditto, 2018).

Summary

Prehospital research, and more broadly health services research, has reached the stage where qualitative research methodologies are widely embraced and their findings and conclusions are being featured in mainstream peer-reviewed medical and health science journals (McLane and Chan, 2018). Practitioners and policy makers see the value of qualitative approaches to research when quantitative methods are unable to find complete or useful answers to difficult and wicked problems that characterise the challenges that the health sector generally and prehospital settings in particular face.

This chapter has provided an introduction to the common characteristics of qualitative research, outlined the strengths and limitations of qualitative research, touched on data collection and analysis and addressed questions of rigour in qualitative research. While the emerging quality criteria are particularly important within the health sector, it needs to be acknowledged that qualitative research is made up of a broad set of methodologies that have long been applied across well-established disciplines. Prehospital practitioners and policy makers need to understand that qualitative research is judged on its own terms within the context of the specific setting and the research questions being asked. To this end, they need to have a basic knowledge and appreciation of the philosophical underpinnings of the research methods being employed and the epistemological stance of the researcher.

The examples of prehospital qualitative research highlighted in this chapter were selected to illustrate the underpinnings of qualitative research methods and how they are increasingly being applied in prehospital settings either as stand-alone approaches or in combination with other research methodologies. A strong characteristic of the examples selected is the preponderance of graduate research student examples cited from across several disciplines and countries.

Across a number of countries, this chapter illustrates that prehospital qualitative researchers are finding creative and innovative ways to answer difficult research questions. These questions often relate to the universal health challenges that we face, such as those related to aging populations and advances in medical technology, that result in growing demand while resources remain limited. In addition, there are challenges associated with both structural and cultural change within society and our healthcare systems associated with changes in cultural diversity, human rights obligations and ethical frameworks, as well as the rise of patient-centred care, that are changing the relationships between health professionals and the community.

Further Reading

Cooper, S. and Endacott, R. 2007. Generic qualitative research: A design for qualitative research in emergency care? *Emergency Medicine Journal*, 24, 816–819.

Kitto, S. C., Chesters, J. and Grbich, C. 2008. Quality in qualitative research. *Medical Journal of Australia*, 188, 243–246.

Mays, N. and Pope, C. 2020. Quality in qualitative research. *In:* Pope, C. and Mays, N. (Eds.) *Qualitative Research in Health Care.* John Wiley and Sons Ltd, Chichester.

McLane, P. and Chan, T. 2018. Stories, voices, and explanations: How qualitative methods may help augment emergency medicine research. *Canadian Journal of Emergency Medicine*, 20, 491–492.

Moore, H. L. and Sanders, T. (Eds.) 2014. *Anthropology in Theory: Issues in Epistemology.* Oxford, Wiley Blackwell.

Morse, J. M. 2015. Critical analysis of strategies for determining rigor in qualitative inquiry. *Qualitative Health Research*, 25, 1212–1222.

Orb, A., Eisenhauer, L. and Wynaden, D. 2001. Ethics in qualitative research. *Journal of Nursing Scholarship*, 33, 93–96.

Sanjari, M. et al. 2014. Ethical challenges of researchers in qualitative studies: The necessity to develop a specific guideline. *Journal of Medical Ethics and History of Medicine*, 7.

Tong, A., Sainsbury, P., and Craig, J. 2007. Consolidated criteria for reporting qualitative research (COREQ): A 32-item checklist for interviews and focus groups. *International Journal for Quality in Health Care*, 19, 349–357.

References

Aldiabat, K. and Navenec, L. 2011. Clarification of the blurred boundaries between grounded theory and ethnography: Differences and similarities. *Turkish Online Journal of Qualitative Inquiry*, 2, 1–13.

Anaf, S. and Sheppard, L. A. 2007. Describing physiotherapy interventions in an emergency department setting: an observational pilot study. *Accident and Emergency Nursing*, 15, 34–39.

Angland, S., Dowling, M. and Casey, D. 2014. Nurses' perceptions of the factors which cause violence and aggression in the emergency department: a qualitative study. *International Emergency Nursing*, 22, 134–139.

Baker, C., Wuest, J. and Stern, P. N. 1992. Method slurring: The grounded theory/phenomenology example. *Journal of Advanced Nursing*, 17, 1355–1360.

Bell, K. 2014. Resisting commensurability: Against informed consent as an anthropological virtue. *American Anthropologist*, 116, 511–522.

Bornstein, E. 2007. Harmonic dissonance: reflections on dwelling in the field. *Ethnos*, 72, 483–508.

Braun, V. and Clarke, V. 2006. Using thematic analysis in psychology. *Qualitative Research in Psychology*, 3, 77–101.

Campeau, A. 2008a. Why paramedics require 'theories-of-practice'. *Journal of Primary Health Care*, 6, Article No. 990296.

Campeau, A. 2008b. The space-control theory of paramedic scene-management. *Symbolic Interaction*, 31, 285–302.

Campeau, A. 2009. Introduction to the 'space-control theory of paramedic scene management'. *Emergency Medicine Journal*, 26, 213–216.

Charmaz, K. 2014. *Constructing Grounded Theory*. Sage, London.

Clarkson, G. 2014. No echo in the ghetto: lived experiences of gay and lesbian paramedics in Australia. Victoria University.

Cooper, S. and Endacott, R. 2007. Generic qualitative research: a design for qualitative research in emergency care? *Emergency Medicine Journal*, 24, 816–819.

Cooper, S., Endacott, R. and Chapman, Y. 2009. Qualitative research: specific designs for qualitative research in emergency care? *Emergency Medicine Journal*, 26, 773–776.

Creswell, J. W. and Poth, C. N. 2016. *Qualitative Inquiry and Research Design: Choosing among five approaches*. Sage, London.

Devenish, A. S. 2014. *Experiences in becoming a paramedic: a qualitative study examining the professional socialisation of university qualified paramedics*. Queensland University of Technology, Australia.

Devenish, S. and O'Meara, P. 2010. Sir Neville Howse (VC), Private John Simpson Kirkpatrick and Private Martin O'Meara (VC) and their contributions to Australian military medicine. *Australasian Journal of Paramedicine*, 8. doi: 10.33151/ajp.8.1.106.

Duneier, M. 2000. Race and peeing on Sixth Avenue. *In:* Twine, F. W. and Warren J. W. (Eds.) *Racing Research, Researching Race: Methodological Dilemmas in Critical Race Studies*, 215–226. New York: New York University Press.

Eberle, T. S. 2015. Exploring another's subjective life-world: A phenomenological approach. *Journal of Contemporary Ethnography*, 44, 563–579.

Endacott, R. et al. 2011. Improving emergency care pathways: an action research approach. *Emergency Medicine Journal*, 28, 203–207.

Evans-Pritchard, E. E. 1937. *Witchcraft, Oracles and Magic Among the Azande*. Clarendon Press, Oxford.

Fassin, D. 2006. The end of ethnography as collateral damage of ethical regulation? *American Ethnologist*, 33, 522–524.

Flick, U. 2018. *Doing Grounded Theory*. Sage, London.

Flood, A. 2010. Understanding phenomenology. *Nurse Researcher*, 17, 7–15.

Forero, R. et al. 2018. Application of four-dimension criteria to assess rigour of qualitative research in emergency medicine. *BMC Health Services Research*, 18, 120.

Furness, S. 2018. Walking in paramedicine: An ontological inquiry. Bendigo, La Trobe University.

Geertz, C. 1973. *The Interpretation of Cultures*. Basic Books, New York.

Glaser, B. and Strauss, A. L. 1966. *Awareness of Dying*. Routledge, New York.

Glaser, B. and Strauss, A. 1967. *Discovery of Grounded Theory: Strategies for qualitative research.* London, Weidenfeld and Nicolson.

Goodwin, D., Mays, N. and Pope, C. 2020. Ethical Issues in Qualitative Research. *Qualitative Research in Health Care*, 27–41.

Gordon, J., Sheppard, L. A. and Anaf, S. 2010. The patient experience in the emergency department: a systematic synthesis of qualitative research. *International emergency nursing*, 18, 80–88.

Harris, M. 1976. History and significance of the emic/etic distinction. *Annual Review of Anthropology*, 5, 329–350.

Hartley, P. R. 2012. Paramedic practice and the cultural and religious needs of pre-hospital patients in Victoria. Victoria University, Australia.

Heidegger, M. 1962. *Being and Time* (J. Macquarrie and E. Robinson, trans.). Harper & Row, New York.

Hickson, H., O'Meara, P. and Huggins, C. 2014. Engaging in community conversation: A means to improving the paramedic student clinical placement experience. *Action Research*, 12, 410–425.

High, H. 2011. Melancholia and anthropology. *American Ethnologist*, 38, 217–233.

Holloway, I. and Todres, L. 2003. The status of method: flexibility, consistency and coherence. *Qualitative Research*, 3, 345–357.

Husserl, E. 1970. *Logical investigations: vols I and II* (J. N. Findlay, trans.). New York, Humanities Press (German original, 1900).

Ingham, G., O'Meara, P., Fry, J. and Crothers, N. 2014. GP supervisors-an investigation into their motivations and teaching activities. *Australian Family Physician*, 43, 808.

Iqbal, M., Spaight, P. A. and Siriwardena, A. N. 2013. Patients' and emergency clinicians' perceptions of improving pre-hospital pain management: a qualitative study. *Emergency Medicine Journal*, 30, e18–e18.

Kalu, F. A. and Bwalya, J. C. 2017. What makes qualitative research good research? An exploratory analysis of critical elements. *International Journal of Social Science Research*, 5, 43–56.

Katz, J. and Csordas, T. J. 2003. Phenomenological ethnography in sociology and anthropology. *Ethnography*, 4, 275–288.

Lambert, V., Glacken, M. and Mccarron, M. 2011. Employing an ethnographic approach: key characteristics. *Nurse Researcher*, 19, 17–24.

Lingard, L., Albert, M., Levinson, W. 2008. Grounded theory, mixed methods, and action research. *British Medical Journal*, 337, a567.

Llewellyn, C. H. 2017. The symbiotic relationship between operational military medicine, tactical medicine, and wilderness medicine: a view through a personal lens. *Wilderness & Environmental Medicine*, 28, S6–S11.

Long, D. N. 2017. *Out of the silo: A qualitative study of paramedic transition to a specialist role in community paramedicine*. Queensland University of Technology, Queensland.

Maguire, B. J. et al. 2018. Preventing EMS workplace violence: A mixed-methods analysis of insights from assaulted medics. *Injury*, 49, 1258–1265.

Malinowski, B. 1922. A*rgonauts of the Western Pacific: An Account of Native Enterprise and Adventure in the Archipelagoes of Melanesian New Guinea*. EP Dutton & Co. Inc, New York.

Markee, N. 2013. Emic and etic in qualitative research. *In:* Chappelle, C. A. (Ed.) *The Encyclopedia of Applied Linguistics*, 1–4. Wiley-Blackwell, Chichester.

Mclane, P. and Chan, T. 2018. Stories, voices, and explanations: How qualitative methods may help augment emergency medicine research. *Canadian Journal of Emergency Medicine*, 20, 491–492.

McManamny, T. et al. 2015. Mixed methods and its application in prehospital research: A systematic review. *Journal of Mixed Methods Research*, 9, 214–231.

Morse, J. M. 2015. Critical analysis of strategies for determining rigor in qualitative inquiry. *Qualitative Health Research*, 25, 1212–1222.

National Association of EMS Physicians and National Association of State EMS Officials 2010. Medical Direction for Operational Emergency Medical Services Programs. *Prehospital Emergency Care*, 14, 544.

Nelson Mandela Foundation (NMF) 2009. *Community Conversations. Communities embracing each other*. South Africa: Nelson Mandela Foundation.

Newton, A. 2011. Specialist practice for paramedics: a bright future. *Journal of Paramedic Practice*, 3, 58–61.

Newton, A. 2012. The ambulance service: the past, present and future. *Journal of Paramedic Practice*, 4, 365–368.

Newton, A. 2014. Ambulance service 2030: The future of paramedics, University of Hertfordshire, Hertfordshire.

Newton, A. and Harris, G. 2015. Leadership and system thinking in the modern ambulance service. *In:* Wankhade, P. and Mackway-Jones, K. (eds.) *Ambulance Services: Leadership and Management Perspectives.* Cham, Springer International Publishing.

O'Meara, D. C. 2020. *Disciplining the Heart: Love, School, and Growing Up Karen in Mae Hong Son.* The Australian National University, Canberra.

O'Meara, P., Tourle, V. and Rae, J. 2012a. Factors influencing the successful integration of ambulance volunteers and first responders into ambulance services. *Health Social Care Community*, 20, 488–496.

O'Meara, P. et al. 2012b. Extending the paramedic role in rural Australia: a story of flexibility and innovation. *Rural & Remote Health*, 12, 1–13.

O'Meara, P., Hickson, H. and Huggins, C. 2014. Starting the conversation: What are the issues for Paramedic student clinical education? *Australasian Journal of Paramedicine*, 11, Article 1.

O'Meara, P., Wingrove, G. and McKeage, M. 2018. Self-regulation and medical direction: Conflicted approaches to monitoring and improving the quality of clinical care in paramedic services. *International Journal of Health Governance*, 23, 233–242.

O'Meara, P., Wingrove, G. and Nolan, M. 2017. Clinical leadership in paramedic services: a narrative synthesis. *International Journal of Health Governance*, 22, 251–268.

Peditto, K. 2018. Reporting qualitative research: Standards, challenges, and implications for health design. *HERD: Health Environments Research & Design Journal*, 11, 16–19.

Pike, K. L. 1967. *Language in Relation to a Unified Theory of the Structure of Human Behavior.* De Gruyter Mouton, Berlin.

Rasku, T. et al. 2020. Community nurse-paramedics' sphere of practice in primary care: an ethnographic study, *BMC Health Services Research*, 21, 710.

Reynolds, L. 2008. Beyond the front line: An interpretative ethnography of an ambulance service, University of South Australia, Adelaide.

Reynolds, L. 2009. Contextualising paramedic culture, in *Paramedics in Australia: contemporary challenges of practice*, edited by P. O'Meara, P. and C. Grbich. Pearson Education Australia, Sydney.

Sanjari, M. et al. 2014. Ethical challenges of researchers in qualitative studies: The necessity to develop a specific guideline. *Journal of Medical Ethics and History of Medicine*, 7, 14.

Stacey, C. L. et al. 2019. Revisiting 'awareness contexts' in the 21st century hospital: How fragmented and specialized care shape patients' Awareness of Dying. *Social Science & Medicine*, 220, 212–218.

Starks, H. and Brown Trinidad, S. 2007. Choose your method: A comparison of phenomenology, discourse analysis, and grounded theory. *Qualitative Health Research*, 17, 1372–1380.

Stone-Resneck, D. 2010. *Community Conversations*. Melbourne, Indigenous Leadership Network, Victoria.

Strathern, M. 2006. Don't eat unwashed lettuce. *American Ethnologist*, 33, 532–534.

Teherani, A. et al. 2015. Choosing a qualitative research approach. *Journal of graduate medical education*, 7, 669–670.

Timmermans, S. and Tavory, I. 2007. Advancing ethnographic research through grounded theory practice. *Handbook of grounded theory*, 493, 513.

Tong, A. et al. 2012. Enhancing transparency in reporting the synthesis of qualitative research: ENTREQ. *BMC Medical Research Methodology*, 12, 181.

Tong, A., Sainsbury, P. and Craig, J. 2007. Consolidated criteria for reporting qualitative research (COREQ): a 32-item checklist for interviews and focus groups. *International Journal for Quality in Health Care*, 19, 349–357.

Urquhart, C. 2019. Grounded theory's best kept secret: The ability to build theory. *In*: Bryant, A. and Charmaz, K. (Eds.) *The SAGE Handbook of Current Developments in Grounded Theory, 89–106*. Sage, London.

Venkatesh, S. 2002. Doin' the Hustle' Constructing the Ethnographer in the American Ghetto. *Ethnography*, 3, 91–111.

Whitehead, D., Taket, A. and Smith, P. 2003. Action research in health promotion. *Health Education Journal*, 62, 5–22.

Williams, J. 2006. Street homelessness: people's experiences of health and health care provision. King's College London, London.

Wojnar, D. M. and Swanson, K. M. 2007. Phenomenology: an exploration. *Journal of Holistic Nursing*, 25, 172–180.

Chapter 7
Mixed Methods Research

Alicia O'Cathain

Chapter Objectives

This chapter will cover:

- The definition of mixed methods research
- The rationale for undertaking mixed methods research in this context
- The different mixed methods designs
- Comparison of the ways of integrating qualitative and quantitative findings
- How to assess the quality of mixed methods research
- How to report and publish mixed methods research
- Common research paradigms for mixed methods research
- How to synthesise evidence in mixed systematic reviews

Introduction

Mixed methods research is where there is at least one quantitative method (quantitative data collection with statistical analysis), and one qualitative method (qualitative data collection with thematic analysis), in the same study. Definitions of mixed methods research vary, with some scholars requiring **integration** of qualitative and quantitative data or findings if the label 'mixed methods research' is to be used. In the definition used in this chapter, integration is not essential but undertaking integration is a sign of a good-quality mixed methods study (O'Cathain et al., 2008). Sometimes researchers use the term 'multi-method' or '**multiple methods**' to describe using quantitative and qualitative methods in the same study where little or no integration is undertaken. For example, an exploration of the use of electronic health records in ambulances used the description 'multiple methods' (Porter et al., 2020). In this chapter, 'mixed methods' is the preferred description of studies combining qualitative and quantitative methods regardless of the amount of integration undertaken. The terms 'multi-method' or 'multiple methods' can be used to describe a study with a number of quantitative methods in it, such as survey and analysis of records, or a number of qualitative methods, such as focus groups and individual semi-structured interviews.

> *Question: How can you tell the difference between a multi-method and mixed methods study?*

Mixed methods research is used when studying prehospital care. A **systematic review** of mixed methods research in prehospital care identified 23 studies published between 2000 and 2012, 18 of them published since 2006 (McManamny et al., 2014). The authors concluded that at the time of their review the use of mixed methods research was relatively new in this field and that prehospital researchers should continue to undertake high-quality mixed methods studies. In this chapter, a number of methodological issues are addressed that prehospital researchers may wish to consider when designing, undertaking and reporting mixed methods research:

- Rationale for using mixed methods research
- Drawing on methodology
- Study designs
- Integration of qualitative and quantitative data and findings
- Articulating **research paradigms**
- Attending to quality
- Reporting and publishing
- Synthesising evidence from mixed methods research
- Challenges in mixed methods research in prehospital care.

Rationale for Using Mixed Methods Research

A key justification for undertaking mixed methods research is that healthcare is complex, and therefore the types of research questions to be addressed are diverse. It sometimes feels necessary to use a combination of qualitative and quantitative research to address the diversity of questions relevant to a topic, and thereby offer a more comprehensive understanding of the issue under study. Indeed this is the rationale put forward in the systematic review of mixed methods research in prehospital care (McManamny et al., 2014).

Quantitative and qualitative methods have strengths for addressing different types of research questions. These research questions include the need to understand how patients experience specific health conditions or treatments, whether new or existing treatments are effective or cost-effective and how different workforce configurations affect the feasibility and quality of healthcare delivery. Quantitative methods best address questions around measurement, such as the prevalence of an attitude or of use of specific treatments, or the size of effect of a treatment. Qualitative methods best address 'how' and 'why' questions, such as how a treatment is delivered in practice, or why patients feel that a new treatment is acceptable or not. Sometimes it is appropriate to address two or more research questions in a single study because they are linked to each other and it feels appropriate to focus on them together. If some questions in a study are best addressed by quantitative methods, and others by qualitative methods, then mixed methods research is required.

Like other research fields, the rationale for mixed methods research is not always articulated explicitly in prehospital care research publications. In a systematic review of mixed methods research in prehospital care, 65% of researchers did not offer a rationale, although the implicit rationale was identified as the need for comprehensiveness in a complex environment (McManamny et al., 2014).

> Question: How would you articulate the rationale for your mixed methods study?

Drawing on Methodology

Methodology is about how research is undertaken. Scholars have written excellent books on how to undertake mixed methods research. Some books offer a detailed overview of why and how to undertake high-quality mixed methods research (Creswell and Plano Clark, 2017), and some offer a workbook approach that takes readers through each step in undertaking a mixed methods study (Fetters, 2019). Studying this methodology can improve the quality of research undertaken. This methodology is considered in the rest of the chapter.

Study Designs

There are different mixed methods research designs. The timing of methods within a study is the most commonly articulated characteristic of a design, with methods used sequentially (one after the other) or concurrently (at the same time).

Sequential Designs

Sequential designs are more common in prehospital research than **concurrent designs** (61% versus 39%) (McManamny et al., 2014). In his early work, Creswell distinguishes between a sequential explanatory design (the qualitative research is undertaken after the quantitative research) and a sequential exploratory design (the qualitative research is undertaken before a quantitative method) (Creswell, 2003). These are very common specific mixed methods designs and have both been used in prehospital research.

Tate and colleagues (2017) undertook a sequential explanatory design when exploring how language can be a barrier to prehospital care provision in South Africa and the USA. They undertook a survey of ambulance personnel followed by an interview study of ambulance personnel. Their rationale for doing the survey first was to identify the range of language barriers and strategies to deal with them, and then examine some of these in greater depth in qualitative interviews. An alternative approach could have been to undertake interviews first to understand what barriers and strategies might exist and then undertake a survey to identify the prevalence of barriers and strategies to deal with them. When deciding on the order of methods, researchers need to think about what is best for their situation. Tate and colleagues (2017) were able to draw on questionnaires used in previous research to develop the questionnaire for their survey, so did not feel that they needed to undertake qualitative research to help them to develop their questionnaire. This specific design has been described in detail (Ivankova et al., 2006).

Wallgren and colleagues (2017) undertook a sequential exploratory design to explore presentations of patients with sepsis in a prehospital setting in Sweden. They started with a review of the narrative sections of ambulance records to identify key words associated with sepsis presentations. They labelled this qualitative research because they used maximum variation sampling when selecting records, sampled records until they reached data saturation and undertook a content analysis of the text within each record. They reflected on why they did not use qualitative interviews with patients or ambulance personnel for this part of the study. They felt that severely ill patients or those with altered mental states would be excluded, and that ambulance personnel have difficulty identifying sepsis. For their quantitative component they identified the frequency of the terms in a large sample of ambulance records.

Some researchers do not use the terms 'exploratory' or 'explanatory' in their design, and this is perfectly acceptable. Indeed, more recent methodological reflections use broader terms to describe designs (Creswell and Plano Clark, 2017). For example, Duncan and colleagues (2018) used the term 'sequential design' when they undertook a qualitative interview study followed by a national prevalence survey of ambulance patients to explore impaired awareness of hypoglycaemia in ambulance service attendances.

A combination of a survey and qualitative interviews is often used in a sequential design, as seen in the examples described here. This combination can be used to explore a topic or to develop a questionnaire or **outcome** measure. In particular, qualitative interviews or focus groups can be used to generate the content and language of a questionnaire to ensure it is both relevant and comprehensible to potential respondents.

Concurrent Designs

Concurrent designs are where two methods are undertaken at the same time. Sometimes these are called **triangulation**, convergent or parallel designs. They are less commonly used in health services research generally (O'Cathain et al., 2007) and in prehospital research (McManamny et al., 2014). They are likely to be used when evaluating interventions where an outcome, process and economic evaluation may be taken concurrently. Outcomes can be measured using **randomised**

controlled trials. For example, Perkins and colleagues (2018) undertook a randomised controlled trial of epinephrine in prehospital cardiac arrest. Because they were evaluating a drug rather than a complex intervention, they did not undertake a process evaluation alongside this trial. Where an intervention is complex, that is, has multiple interacting components (Craig et al., 2008), it is recommended that process evaluations are undertaken concurrently with the outcome evaluations (Moore et al., 2014). These process evaluations are often mixed methods. They explore the context in which the intervention was implemented, how the intervention delivered benefit (sometimes called mechanisms of action), the feasibility and acceptability of the intervention and how it was delivered in practice. Some process evaluations are qualitative only, consisting of interviews with staff who deliver the intervention, interviews with patients receiving the intervention and sometimes non-participant observation of the intervention being delivered. An example of this is an evaluation of new protocols for paramedics to assess older people after a fall (Snooks et al., 2017). This was a complex intervention because it had multiple interacting components including an assessment protocol, referral pathways, a falls service and training for paramedics. Outcomes were measured in a large randomised controlled trial. A qualitative study was undertaken alongside the trial. This consisted of interviews with patients who had used the new pathway to explore their experiences, and with paramedics and managers to explore how the intervention had been implemented.

Sometimes quasi-experimental or non-randomised designs are used in the outcome evaluation. An example is a mixed methods evaluation of motorbike ambulances in rural Sierra Leone for maternal care (Bhopal et al., 2013). The focus of this study was the use, acceptability and accessibility of the new service rather than its effectiveness or cost-effectiveness. The quantitative research used ambulance records to identify numbers using the service. The qualitative research involved focus groups in rural communities to explore the acceptability and accessibility of this new service.

Using More Than Two Methods in a Design

Sometimes designs include more than two methods, using a number of methods in different phases. It is difficult to find a label to describe these more complex designs. It is best to describe the design by showing the timing of different components and explaining how they relate to each other. For example, a mixed methods study of variation in ambulance non-conveyance rates consisted of three phases (O'Cathain et al., 2018b). The study was undertaken because different regional ambulances services in England had very different rates of calls ending in telephone advice only (sometimes called 'hear and treat', where callers are referred to an onsite clinician who offers them self-care advice or advice about contacting alternatives to sending an ambulance). There was also variation in rates of calls that were discharged at scene (sometimes called 'see and treat', where an ambulance is dispatched but the patient is treated on scene and not conveyed to hospital). The first phase of the study was a qualitative interview study of managers, paramedics and healthcare commissioners for each of the ten large regional ambulance services in England to understand their perceptions of determinants of non-conveyance within each ambulance service (Knowles et al.,

2018). In the second phase, there were three concurrent studies. Two of them were quantitative and involved the analysis of electronically available routine data from ambulance services. Routine data from ten ambulance services were combined and used to test determinants of variation in non-conveyance (O'Cathain et al., 2018a). The other quantitative dataset was routine data from one ambulance service only and involved linking data from the ambulance service, emergency departments and a national mortality dataset to identify the appropriateness of the two types of non-conveyance (Coster et al., 2019). The third study in this phase was a qualitative study that used non-participant observation and interviews to explore variation in calls offered telephone advice (O'Hara et al., 2019). The third phase involved a mixed methods study of non-conveyance for breathing difficulties, bringing together all the data about calls to ambulance services from the different datasets in the earlier phases and focusing on this common reason for calling an emergency ambulance.

Drawing a Diagram of a Study Design

A diagram of the design can help to explain simple or complex designs to readers. Diagrams can take different formats by simply showing the methods used and the timing of those methods. More complex diagrams can show the timing of data collection, analysis and integration. Examples of diagrams are available in prehospital research (O'Cathain et al., 2018b; Tate et al., 2017).

> **Question:** *How would you draw a diagram of your study – would you include when the analysis took place?*

Other Ways of Describing Designs

Sometimes researchers draw attention to the priority or dominance of different methods within a study, labelling a study as 'qualitatively dominant' if the survey undertaken prior to a qualitative study is mainly there to help identify a rich sample for the qualitative study (Tate et al., 2017). A design might also be described as dominant if most of the research questions and resources focus on one methodology. For example, most of the components of a mixed methods study of developing new ways of measuring the quality and impact of ambulance service care were quantitative (Turner et al., 2019). Only one component used qualitative research; this explored patients' perspectives of outcomes important to them (Togher et al., 2015). A lot of mixed methods studies give equal weight to the qualitative and the quantitative components, so researchers usually only point out where there is dominance. A review of 23 mixed methods research studies in prehospital care identified that 22% were predominantly qualitative, 35% were predominantly quantitative and 43% had equal weight (McManamny et al., 2014).

Methods Used Within Designs

Quantitative methods commonly used in prehospital research to date include surveys (21%) and reviews of routine records (16%). Common qualitative methods include face-to-face interviews (21%), non-participant observation (10%) and focus groups (8%) (McManamny et al., 2014).

Closed and Open Questions on Questionnaires

There is a lack of clarity about the best label to apply when using closed and open questions on a questionnaire in a survey. Some mixed methods scholars would not label this mixed methods, because there is only one method used – a survey – and the rich description associated with qualitative research is rarely available in short narrative text offered on questionnaires. Other scholars would view this combination as mixed methods research because both numerical and text data are collected, and each is analysed differently. A number of prehospital researchers have labelled this approach as mixed methods research. For example, Sinclair and colleagues (2018) describe their study of self-reporting of safety incidents by paramedics as mixed methods research; closed and open questions were used in their survey. Bigham and colleagues (2014) use a similar approach to explore self-reported exposure to violence in the prehospital workplace but call this a 'mixed methods cross-sectional survey'. This is a better description because it is clear that a single method – a survey – has been used. Pyper and Paterson (2016) also use the term 'mixed methods survey' when exploring fatigue and mental health in ambulance personnel in Australia.

Integration of Qualitative and Quantitative Data and Findings

Integration is the relationship, links or interaction between different components in a mixed methods study. Integration is important because attending to it ensures that the whole is more than the sum of the parts, increasing the yield of insights from a study (O'Cathain et al., 2010). Integration is built into some study designs. For example, the results of a survey may help identify the sample for a qualitative interview component, a sample that might otherwise have been difficult to obtain. Or qualitative interviews may help to identify the content of a questionnaire for a survey so that its yield is greater because it is highly relevant to the sample. Even though integration is often built into sequential designs, further integration is possible and often beneficial. Integration is not built into concurrent designs and therefore researchers need to make extra efforts to undertake integration. Techniques for integration have been identified in healthcare research and other disciplines (Fetters, 2019; O'Cathain et al., 2010).

'Triangulation protocol' is a really useful integration technique (Farmer et al., 2006). This was devised for bringing together findings from different qualitative components of a study but has been adapted for use in mixed methods research (O'Cathain et al., 2010). The first step is to analyse the qualitative and quantitative components of a study separately. The second step is to identify a set of themes relevant to both sets of findings. This is partly a deductive process, drawing on the research objectives or a relevant conceptual framework for the topic under study, and partly inductive, drawing on the findings of each study component. The third step is to display all the findings related to an issue/theme on the same page in a grid/matrix/joint display and consider the relationships between findings from different components. The authors of this approach recommend that researchers consider agreement, partial agreement, dissonance and silence between findings from different components

(Farmer et al., 2006). In mixed methods research, it is more useful to consider: agreement/convergence; complementarity rather than 'partial agreement', thinking about how the findings from one method help to explain or illuminate those of another; disagreement/dissonance; and silence, where there are no relevant findings from one component when these findings might be expected. The analyst is aiming to draw '**meta-inferences**' from this process, that is, conclusions that encompass the different components of a mixed methods study. A detailed example of using triangulation protocol in prehospital research has been published for a study of variation in ambulance non-conveyance, where findings from five study components were considered (O'Cathain et al., 2018b). See **Box 7.1** for a step-by-step guide to how this integration occurred.

A triangulation protocol grid is one way of making a 'joint display' to facilitate integration in mixed methods research (Guetterman et al., 2015). Guetterman and colleagues (2015) offer a number of examples of these joint displays in their paper. Joint displays can be used to display data, as well as findings, from different components of a study. For example, when a survey questionnaire is completed by someone who has also been interviewed, their data can be put side by side and compared. Data can be displayed in a matrix where the rows are cases and the columns are data from different data collection methods for each case. Researchers then look for patterns within and across these cases.

Box 7.1 Describing the Use of a Joint Display to Facilitate Integration in the Variation in Ambulance Non-conveyance (VAN) Study

It is helpful to look at the integration grid constructed for the VAN study, displayed in the open access final study report (O'Cathain et al., 2018b). The following steps were taken to construct this grid:

1. The methods/components of two of the three phases of this study became the columns in the integration grid:

   a. Qualitative interview study of staff perceptions of non-conveyance within their ambulance service (ten ambulance services)

   b. Analysis of routine data on rates of non-conveyance from ten ambulance services

   c. Analysis of 24-hour recontact rates from ten ambulance services

   d. Analysis of data from one ambulance service linked to mortality and subsequent service use

   e. Qualitative study of telephone advice as the final outcome in three ambulance services.

The third phase used these five datasets to focus on the specific symptom of 'breathing difficulties', so this phase was excluded from the integration process, which focused on non-conveyance for any symptom.

2. Consideration was then given to constructing the themes in the rows of the grid. Appleby's framework of causes of variation in healthcare (Appleby et al., 2011) had been used as a conceptual framework for the study. Consideration was given to using this framework to structure the rows/themes. However, it only captured some of the key issues specific to prehospital care so an inductive process was used akin to a thematic analysis in qualitative research where themes and sub-themes are identified. Findings from each component were read and a set of themes and sub-themes identified that encompassed all the findings. Appleby's framework was helpful in structuring these themes. These were labelled as 'factors' rather than themes, and 'aspects of factors' rather than sub-themes, because an aim of the study had been to identify factors affecting variation in non-conveyance. Factors included: data inaccuracy, random variation, patients' characteristics (patients' expectations, morbidity, demographics, rurality), commissioning priorities, call characteristics (time of day, source as NHS111 or other), workforce (shortages, skill mix, how workforce used, staff morale, length of service), software, organisation characteristics (stability, motivation to undertake non-conveyance), wider healthcare system (provision of services, connectivity with services, pressure in the healthcare system, complexity of the healthcare system), national issues (response-time targets, volume of calls), safety and appropriateness.

3. The findings from each component were written in the grid for each 'factor' and 'aspects of a factor'. These summary statements were kept short to allow for easy comparison across components.

4. Then the lead researcher read the findings for each 'aspect of a factor' and considered whether they converged, complemented each other, disagreed or there was unexpected silence. Then they wrote a conclusion or 'meta-inference' about that factor. Farmer and colleagues (2006) recommend that two researchers do this independently and compare notes. With a deadline looming for submitting the report to the funder, the lead researcher decided to do this alone and made this clear when reporting the study.

5. Finally, the lead researcher used the column of conclusions to summarise the conclusions of the study. The grid was published in the final report so that it acted as an audit trail for reported conclusions.

Another approach to integration is called 'following a thread' (Moran-Ellis et al., 2006), where hypotheses can be generated from findings from one component of a study and then explored or tested in another component, with the researcher moving backwards and forwards between datasets until they draw conclusions. An example of this is detailed elsewhere (O'Cathain et al., 2010).

Attending to Quality

When using different methods within a study, it is important to attend to the quality criteria associated with each method. That is, any survey should follow guidance on undertaking excellent surveys and any focus groups should follow guidance on undertaking these to a high standard. These quality criteria can also be used by external reviewers of the completed research to draw conclusions about the methodological quality of the study. There are also extra issues to attend to in mixed methods research. Researchers need to ensure they have used a design appropriate to their research question(s) and consider whether any integration has been undertaken well.

A key way to help external reviewers judge the quality of a mixed methods study is to make sure that principal aspects of the study are reported clearly, that is, that transparency is offered. To do this, researchers can follow some short reporting guidance, consisting of six items, called Good Reporting of A Mixed Methods Study (GRAMMS), first reported in O'Cathain et al. (2008) (see **Box 7.2**).

Prehospital researchers wanting to know more about quality in mixed methods research can read a comprehensive assessment of ways to address quality (O'Cathain, 2010), including a discussion of the applicability of transferability rather than **generalisability** to meta-inferences drawn from mixed methods research. Fàbregues and Molina-Azorín (2017) are leading scholars of quality in mixed methods research, offering further up-to-date debate and reflection.

> *Question: How important is the transparency of research to your understanding of quality? Are you aware of the quality criteria for specific methods you are using in your mixed methods study?*

Box 7.2 Good Reporting of a Mixed Methods Study (GRAMMS)

Describe the justification for using a mixed methods approach to the research question.

Describe the design in terms of the purpose, priority and sequence of methods.

Describe each method in terms of sampling, data collection and analysis.

Describe where integration has occurred, how it has occurred and who participated in it.

Describe any limitation of one method associated with the presence of the other method.

Describe any insights gained from mixing or integrating methods.

Articulating Research Paradigms

A paradigm is a set of beliefs. Different academic disciplines in different countries in different decades can have very different beliefs about research and how best to do it. Healthcare researchers have traditionally favoured a **positivist** or **postpositivist** approach where they believe that it is essential that researchers are objective, and that removing **bias** is paramount to good research. They have been interested mainly in research questions that require measurement – such as what proportion of paramedics use a specific protocol, or whether patients who received a new treatment improved more than patients who received a standard treatment. Because they have been interested in measurement, they have used quantitative methods. In recent decades, healthcare researchers have become more interested in a different set of questions, such as why paramedics do not use certain protocols in certain situations, questions that are best addressed using qualitative research. Although qualitative research can be undertaken within a positivist or postpositivist paradigm, it is usually undertaken within a constructivist paradigm where researchers believe that it is not possible to be an objective researcher and that every researcher sees the world through a different lens. This means that reflexivity is an important consideration, that is, researchers consider how their beliefs are affecting any data collection, analysis and interpretation, and reflect on this rather than think they can eliminate it. Quantitative research can also be undertaken within a constructivist paradigm. This means that a mixed methods researcher can undertake their quantitative and qualitative components within a postpositivist or a constructivist paradigm. In healthcare research, it is much more usual for researchers to consider other paradigms such as **pragmatism** when undertaking mixed methods research.

Pragmatism is a common position to adopt in mixed methods research (Creswell and Plano Clark, 2017). It is often described as emphasising the use of methods that work for the research questions, or where the utility of the research is highly valued. This is highly relevant for prehospital researchers where the rationale for undertaking any research is to improve health and healthcare delivery in the prehospital setting. Healthcare researchers rarely discuss their paradigms in journal articles, and the same is true for prehospital researchers. Of 23 studies in a systematic review of mixed methods studies in prehospital care, only two were explicit about their paradigm (McManamny et al., 2014). Even though paradigms are rarely articulated, it is helpful for researchers to consider their beliefs about research so that they can understand why they privilege some methods and quality criteria over others. Prehospital researchers undertaking PhDs are likely to have to be explicit about this in their thesis.

> *Question: Do you believe that researchers need to be objective or can be objective?*

Reporting and Publishing Mixed Methods Research

Outside and within the field of prehospital research, researchers sometimes publish a mixed methods study in a single peer-reviewed journal article (Tate et al., 2017; Wallgren et al., 2017). Sometimes researchers write a mixed methods report (for example, O'Cathain et al., 2018b; Porter et al., 2020; Turner et al., 2019) but then break the study up into its methodological pieces to be published separately in different journal articles. For example, the VAN study described earlier was published in a mixed methods research report with a 50,000 word limit (O'Cathain et al., 2018b). When this study was published in peer-reviewed journals, one journal article focused on the qualitative component of interviews with managers and paramedics discussing what affected non-conveyance in their service (Knowles et al., 2018). Another article reported the quantitative analysis exploring determinants of variation between ambulance services (O'Cathain et al., 2018a). And yet another article reported the qualitative component on how telephone advice was delivered in three of the ambulance services (O'Hara et al., 2019).

This approach of breaking up studies and publishing them separately is understandable because researchers need to report the detailed methods and findings of each component. Sometimes a single journal article may not allow for reporting the necessary detail of more than one component if the word limit is 3,000 words. Even journals available in electronic format with no hard limit on the length of an article may recommend that articles are short to ensure they are easy to read. A problem with breaking a study up into pieces like this is that there may be no opportunity to report the findings emerging from any integration that took place. If a mixed methods journal article is not possible, a way of addressing integration within a mono-method article is to connect the component being reported to the over-arching mixed methods study in the introduction so that readers know it is part of a wider study, and then discuss integration and the relationship with findings from other components in the discussion section of the article. In the VAN study described earlier, Knowles and colleagues' article on the qualitative research highlighted the over-arching mixed methods study in the introduction section, described it briefly in the methods section and then described how the qualitative research was used to inform a statistical regression reported in another article. Because the statistical regression article was published, Knowles and colleagues were able to reference this article and briefly describe the findings, so readers knew the findings of different parts of the study when reading a single journal article.

It is usual to publish the results of full randomised controlled trials and the accompanying process evaluations or qualitative research separately. Price et al. (2020) report the effect of an enhanced Paramedic Acute Stroke Treatment Assessment on thrombolysis delivery, showing that it was not effective in a cluster randomised controlled trial called PASTA. Lally et al. (2020) report the qualitative study of paramedics' views of the feasibility and acceptability of delivering the intervention in the PASTA trial. The context of the qualitative study – the PASTA trial – is described in the abstract of Lally's article and is referenced in the background section. The authors identify some perceived benefits of the intervention and also considerable barriers to its use in practice, explaining the null finding of the trial.

Mixed Methods and Systematic Reviews

Although systematic reviews historically have focused on evidence from randomised controlled trials, reviews that focus on qualitative, quantitative and mixed methods research are increasingly common. They can be called 'mixed reviews' or 'mixed methods systematic reviews' or 'systematic mixed studies reviews' (Hong and Pluye, 2019). Examples in prehospital research include a scoping review to explore patient safety in ambulance services using a 'mixed methods design' (Fisher et al., 2015), a planned systematic review of factors influencing medical errors in the prehospital paramedic environment (Walker et al., 2019) using the Joanna Briggs Institute Methodology for Mixed Methods Reviews (Lizarondo et al., 2017) and a 'systematic mixed studies review' of acute pain management in children in the prehospital setting (Whitley et al., 2021). Authors may only include quantitative and qualitative studies, assessing the quality of each study using methods-specific criteria. When they include mixed methods studies, they can assess the quality of studies using the Mixed Methods Appraisal Tool (MMAT), which pays attention to the mixed methods aspects of a study such as its rationale and integration (Hong et al., 2018). In such reviews, researchers can also add into their synthesis the insights gained from integration of qualitative and quantitative findings.

Challenges of Undertaking Mixed Methods Research in a Prehospital Care Environment

Tate et al. (2017) have reflected on their experiences of using mixed methods research in prehospital care. They identified challenges that are likely to be applicable to any prehospital research, not simply mixed methods research. They reflected on their study of language barriers between ambulance personnel and patients and the effect this had on care in America and South Africa. One challenge they faced was gaining access to undertake research in the different ambulance services in each country because they were external researchers. Prehospital care is stressful and dynamic, and the authors reflected that this might result in a reluctance to open up to researchers in case they are unfairly judged. The authors also noted the need to build relationships early in the planning of the study to build trust between ambulance service management and researchers; they started doing this two years prior to their study. A further challenge they noted was the variation between different organisations and the staffing structures, which made seeking permissions for the research challenging. This study was undertaken in two countries and challenges may differ between countries.

A facilitator of mixed methods research in prehospital care in the future is the number of paramedics undertaking higher degrees, studying mixed methods research as part of their education. This bodes well for paramedics leading their own mixed methods studies to improve health and healthcare in this important healthcare context.

Summary

Mixed methods research is important when using research to understand and improve prehospital care. A single researcher, or a team, needs expertise in both qualitative and quantitative research, and an understanding of the rationales, designs and integration techniques of mixed methods research that allow researchers to maximise their insights about the topic under study.

Further Reading

Fetters, M. D. 2019. *The Mixed Methods Research Workbook: Activities for Designing, Implementing, and Publishing Projects*. London, Sage Publications.

References

Appleby, J et al. 2011. *Variations in Health Care: The Good, the Bad and the Inexplicable*. London, The King's Fund.

Bhopal, S., Haplin, J. S. and Gerein, N. 2013. Emergency obstetric referral in rural Sierra Leone: What can motorbike ambulances contribute? A mixed-methods study. *Maternal and Child Health Journal*, 17, 1038–1043.

Bigham, B. L. et al. 2014. Phd paramedic self-reported exposure to violence in the Emergency Medical Services (EMS) workplace: A mixed-methods cross-sectional survey. *Prehospital Emergency Care*, 18, 489–494.

Coster, J. et al. 2019. Outcomes for patients who contact the emergency ambulance service and are not transported to the emergency department: A data linkage study. *Prehospital Emergency Care*, 23, 566–577.

Craig, P. et al. 2008. Developing and evaluating complex interventions: The new Medical Research Council guidance. *BMJ*, 337, A1655.

Creswell, J. 2003. *Research Design: Qualitative, Quantitative, and Mixed Methods Approaches*, 2nd Edn., Thousand Oaks, Sage.

Creswell, J. and Plano Clark, V. 2017. *Designing and Conducting Mixed Methods Research*, 3rd Edn. London, SAGE Publications.

Duncan, E. A. et al. 2018. Role and prevalence of impaired awareness of hypoglycaemia in ambulance service attendances to people who have had a severe hypoglycaemic emergency: A mixed methods study. *BMJ Open*, 8, E019522.

Fàbregues, S. and Molina-Azorín, J. F. 2017. Addressing quality in mixed methods research: a review and recommendations for a future agenda. *Quality & Quantity: International Journal of Methodology*, 51: 2847–2863.

Farmer, T. et al. 2006. Developing and implementing a triangulation protocol for qualitative health research. *Qualitative Health Research*, 16, 377–394.

Fetters, M. 2019. *The Mixed Methods Research Workbook. Activities For Designing, Implementing, And Publishing Projects*. London, Sage Publications.

Fisher, J. et al. 2015. *Patient Safety in Ambulance Services: A Scoping Review*. Southampton, NIHR Journals Library.

Guetterman, T. C., Fetters, M. D. and Creswell, J. W. 2015. Integrating quantitative and qualitative results in health science mixed methods research through joint displays. *Annals of Family Medicine*, 13, 554–561.

Hong, Q. and Pluye, P. 2019. A conceptual framework for critical appraisal in systematic mixed studies reviews. *Journal of Mixed Methods Research*, 13, 446–460.

Hong, Q. et al. 2018. The Mixed Methods Appraisal Tool (MMAT) version 2018 for information professionals and researchers. *Education For Information*, 34, 285–291.

Ivankova, N., Creswell, J. and Stick, S. 2006. Using mixed-methods sequential explanatory design: From theory to practice. *Field Methods*, 18, 3–20.

Knowles, E., Bishop-Edwards, L. and O'Cathain, A. 2018. Exploring variation in how ambulance services address non-conveyance: A qualitative interview study. *BMJ Open*, 8, E024228.

Lally, J. et al. 2020. Paramedic experiences of using an enhanced stroke assessment during a cluster randomised trial: A qualitative thematic analysis. *Emergency Medicine Journal*, 37, 480–485.

Lizarondo, L., Stern, C. and Carrier, J. 2017. Chapter 8: Mixed methods systematic reviews. *In:* Aromataris, E. and Munn, Z. (Eds.) *Joanna Briggs Institute Reviewer's Manual.* Adelaide, The Joanna Briggs Institute.

Mcmanamny, T. et al. 2014. Mixed methods and its application in prehospital research: A systematic review. *Journal of Mixed Methods*, 9, 214–231.

Moore, G. F. et al. 2014. Process evaluation of complex interventions. Medical Research Council guidance. *BMJ*, 350, H1258.

Moran-Ellis, J. et al. 2006. Triangulation and integration: Processes, claims and implications. *Qualitative Research*, 6, 45–59.

O'Cathain, A. 2010. Assessing the quality of mixed methods research: Toward a comprehensive framework. *In:* Tashakkori, A. and Teddlie, C. (Eds.) *Handbook of Mixed Methods Research*, 2nd Edn. London, Sage.

O'Cathain, A. et al. 2018a. Why do ambulance services have different non-transport rates? A national cross sectional study. *Plos One*, 13, E0204508.

O'Cathain, A. et al. 2018b. Understanding variation in ambulance service non-conveyance rates: A mixed methods study. *Health Services and Delivery Research*, 6, 1–191.

O'Cathain, A., Murphy, E. and Nicholl, J. 2007. Why, and how, mixed methods research is undertaken in health services research: A mixed methods study. *BMC Health Services Research*, 7, 85.

O'Cathain, A., Murphy, E. and Nicholl, J. 2008. The quality of mixed methods studies in health services research. *Journal of Health Services Research and Policy*, 13, 92–98.

O'Cathain, A., Murphy, E. and Nicholl, J. 2010. Three techniques for integrating qualitative and quantitative methods in health services research. *BMJ*, 341, 1147–1150.

O'Hara, R. et al. 2019. Variation in the delivery of telephone advice by emergency medical services: A qualitative study in three services. *BMJ Quality and Safety*, 28, 556–563.

Perkins, G. D. et al. 2018. A randomized trial of epinephrine in out-of-hospital cardiac arrest. *New England Journal of Medicine*, 379, 711–721.

Porter, A. et al. 2020. Electronic health records in ambulances: The ERA multiple-methods study. *Health Services and Delivery Research*, 8, 1–140.

Price, C. I. et al. 2020. Effect of an enhanced paramedic acute stroke treatment assessment on thrombolysis delivery during emergency stroke care. A cluster randomized clinical trial. *JAMA Neurology*, 77, 840–848.

Pyper, Z. and Paterson, J. L. 2016. Fatigue and mental health in Australian rural and regional ambulance personnel. *Emergency Medicine Australasia*, 21, 62–66.

Sinclair, J. E. et al. 2018. Barriers to self-reporting patient safety incidents by paramedics: A mixed methods study. *Prehospital Emergency Care*, 22, 762–772.

Snooks, H. A. et al. 2017. Support and Assessment for Fall Emergency Referrals (SAFER) 2: A cluster randomised trial and systematic review of clinical effectiveness and cost-effectiveness of new protocols for emergency ambulance paramedics to assess older people following a fall with referral to community-based care when appropriate. *Health Technology Assessment*, 21, 1–218.

Tate, R., Hodkinson, P. W. and Sussman, A. L. 2017. Lessons learned from the application of mixed methods to an international study of prehospital language barriers. *Journal of Mixed Methods Research*, 11, 469–486.

Togher, F. J. et al. 2015. Reassurance as a key outcome valued by emergency ambulance service users: A qualitative interview study. *Health Expect*, 18, 2951–2961.

Turner, J. et al. 2019. Developing new ways of measuring the quality and impact of ambulance service care: The PhOEBE mixed-methods research programme. *Programme Grants of Applied Research*, 7, 1–90.

Walker, D. et al. 2019. Contributing factors that influence medication errors in the prehospital paramedic environment: A mixed-method systematic review protocol. *BMJ Open*, 9, E034094.

Wallgren, U. M., Bohm, K. E. M. and Kurland, L. 2017. Presentations of adult septic patients in the prehospital setting as recorded by emergency medical services: A mixed methods analysis. *Scandinavian Journal of Trauma, Resuscitation and Emergency Medicine*, 25, 23.

Whitley, G. A. et al. 2021. The predictors, barriers and facilitators to effective management of acute pain in children by emergency medical services: A systematic mixed studies review. *Journal of Child Health Care*, 25, 481–503.

Chapter 8

Consensus Methods

Aloysius Niroshan Siriwardena and Gregory Adam Whitley

Chapter Objectives

This chapter will cover:

- A definition of what consensus methods are
- The rationale for using consensus methods
- Which research questions are appropriate for a consensus method
- An explanation of the main consensus designs
- Detailed description of the Delphi process, nominal group technique and consensus development conference
- Comparing and contrasting of the different consensus methods
- Examples of consensus methods

Introduction

To achieve consensus involves people coming to an agreement about something. **Consensus methods** involve a set of scientific methods designed to enable a group of people with relevant knowledge to reach agreement on policy or decision making in an area of uncertainty.

The three commonest consensus study designs are the **Delphi method**, the **nominal group technique** and the **consensus development conference** (Bowling, 2009). Sometimes, one or more of these methods can be modified or combined to enable consensus to be reached on a particular topic.

The use of consensus methods in healthcare developed in the second half of the 20th century as a way of applying formal techniques to achieve agreement on best practice in clinical care. They have been expanded to prioritise other aspects of importance to health policy makers, researchers, educators, organisations and practitioners. Soliciting opinions from a group rather than a single expert is considered to have the advantage of incorporating a range of opinions, where the opinions of knowledgeable individuals may differ, rather than relying on the opinion of a single expert, but it comes with the disadvantages inherent in any group process.

This chapter will describe the definition of consensus methods, explore the rationale for using them, classify different consensus designs, discuss which research questions are most appropriate for such methods and examine how to select participants for consensus exercises. We also discuss the potential drawbacks of consensus methods in general and some specific examples. Finally, we will present examples of how consensus designs have been used in the prehospital field.

Definition of and Rationale for Consensus Methods

Consensus methods are formal systematic research designs for groups to reach agreement, where possible, on areas of uncertainty.

Consensus designs have and can be used for a variety of research questions, particularly when other types of research method are unable or inappropriate to answer these questions. Examples in the prehospital research field include prioritising the most important research questions (Snooks et al., 2009), agreeing best practice in reporting research methods or clinical guidelines (https://www.equator-network .org/reporting-guidelines/), ranking the most relevant clinical **outcomes** or indicators (Coster et al., 2018a) or when deciding on appropriate healthcare. In this regard, consensus statements or guidelines have been developed to advise on clinical assessment, investigation, diagnosis or healthcare, particularly when there are gaps in the research evidence. They are also used to produce consensus guidelines for curricula and teaching.

The use of consensus methods to agree consensus guidelines for best practice in clinical diagnosis or treatment, where evidence is lacking, is the commonest use of these techniques but is also arguably the most open to criticism. This is because of problems of deficiencies in evidence (which of course is why they are used in the first place), **bias** in selection and views of participants who may be subject to influences inside and outside the consensus group, the potential for harm from guidelines, the lack of costs attributed to them and the failure to implement recommendations. All of these were neatly summarised over three decades ago by the late Petr Skrabanek in his polemic against consensus guidelines, 'Nonsensus consensus' (Skrabanek, 1990), which as the title suggests attacked their **validity** and **reliability**.

Despite these criticisms, consensus guidelines continue to be produced. Developers have tried to address some of the criticisms by careful selection of a wide range of stakeholders, including lay representatives, by explicitly stating the strength of evidence on which guidelines are based and by considering the potential for harm and costs of recommendations – for example, those from the National Institute for Health and Care Excellence (NICE, 2013).

There are many other types of research questions for which consensus methods are arguably less controversial. These include making decisions on research priorities (Snooks et al., 2009), agreeing the content of an educational curriculum or assessment (Gugiu et al., 2021), determining desirable attributes of EMS clinicians (Kilner, 2004) and prioritising evidence-based quality indicators (Coster et al., 2018a), all of which are relevant to the prehospital field.

Consensus methods are often inconsistently applied, so it is important that the exact details of the method being used are described in detail (Humphrey-Murto et al., 2017).

Consensus Designs

The three main consensus designs – the Delphi method, nominal group technique and consensus development conference – are characterised by features related to how prior information is introduced, how participants are identified and selected, whether they are allowed to meet or remain anonymous, how expertise is shared between them, whether interaction is enabled or not, whether feedback is provided, which individual priorities are sought, which iteration or re-ranking is facilitated and how agreement is achieved.

The selection of participants is a controversial aspect of these methods because of **selection bias** and the possibility that the participants who have been selected or have volunteered might contribute differently or assign different priorities from others. Participants, also termed key informants, are recruited for consensus methods depending on the research question and their expertise or knowledge of the particular question under consideration. They could include academic or policy experts, health professionals, patient contributors or a combination of these different stakeholders, each of whom bring their own perspective to the problem at hand. To what extent and how they are enabled to interact is an important distinguishing feature of the different methods.

Agreement is reached from the opinions solicited, where possible informed through literature reviews, prompts and scenarios or vignettes; through sharing views and feedback that support judgments through rating, ranking, voting or discussion; and through statistical or qualitative aggregation in various combinations, depending on the specific method or modification of the method being used.

Delphi Method

The Delphi process consists of two or more surveys to a group of key informants designed to generate and prioritise ideas. It seeks to overcome the drawbacks of group effects by using anonymity to ensure that opinions are arrived at independently or changed after consideration, using controlled feedback to reduce noise from redundant information, and using statistical analysis of group responses to determine whether a consensus can be reached or not (Brown, 1968; Dalkey, 1967).

Delphi is the name of a place in Ancient Greece thought at the time to be the centre of the world. It was named after a mythical dragon named Delphyne who was slain by the god Apollo. It was where people consulted the oracle, a priestess who according to myth was the mouthpiece of the deity and thus able to predict the future. The Delphi study or process was originally developed in the 1940s and 1950s at the US RAND Corporation to make military predictions, but was extended to forecasting in education and other areas of policy including healthcare.

The Delphi method or process as it was originally conceived was an attempt to gather a range of opinions rather than risk relying on a single possibly flawed opinion, and to overcome the possible group effects of talkative but not necessarily more knowledgeable individuals influencing a group. It also sought to address the problems of experts' reluctance to change their publicly stated opinions, 'noise' from specious or redundant rather than relevant material being introduced to discussions and the 'bandwagon effect' of group pressure to conform or compromise where consensus is absent (Brown, 1968; Dalkey, 1967).

Delphi questionnaire surveys start with broad questions to gather ideas. Subsequent surveys are more focused and consist of rating or ranking priorities, often using Likert scales, related to the question under consideration. At each stage after the first, participants receive feedback on their individual responses and those of the whole group, which helps to inform their subsequent ratings. Median and interquartile ranges of group responses are provided to represent the range of opinion in comparison with the individual group member.

Participants are encouraged to reconsider their ratings, to provide justification for them particularly when they are out of kilter with other members and to critique previous responses and give further information. This can lead to iterative modification of question items, which together with feedback of individual and group ratings encourages convergence. The process often involves three to four rounds of surveys but can be completed after just two or continue beyond four rounds until consensus is achieved for sufficient items (Fink et al., 1984; Jones and Hunter, 1995).

Early modifications of the Delphi process included allowing participants to add further questions which would help to inform others and enable them to reconsider their opinions and estimates, and interviewing participants to learn more about the rationale for their views (Brown, 1968). Other modifications include members meeting to resolve uncertainties (Jones and Hunter, 1995), although this seems to negate the idea of anonymity, which was central to the original idea of the Delphi process.

Using information summaries, prompts and other cues in the context of interviews to check that all relevant information has been considered when making judgements has also been advocated to address problems of cognitive bias such as anchoring or overconfidence (Morgan, 2014). Adjusting the makeup of groups to ensure heterogeneity and using techniques for stimulating conflicting views and debate to increase diversity of opinion have also been advocated to improve the quality of group decisions (Bolger and Wright, 2011).

Reliability increases as the number of participants and rounds rises, but participant fatigue, complexity and costs are drawbacks (Fink et al., 1984). Suggestions for improving the quality of Delphi studies include specifying at the outset how participants will be selected or excluded, whether the objective is to reach consensus or just present a level of agreement and, in the case of the former predetermining how consensus is defined, deciding when items will be discarded and how many rounds the process will continue for before being stopped (Diamond et al., 2014).

Nominal Group Technique

The nominal group technique (NGT), sometimes referred to as the expert panel method, is a structured, facilitated, face-to-face meeting of key informants designed to generate ideas independently, agree a composite list of the most relevant ideas through discussion and refinement in a group or subgroups of participants and then to rate, rank or vote to prioritise the ideas put forward, in two (or sometimes more) rounds to achieve a consensus. The technique, developed by Delbecq and Van de Ven in the USA in the 1960s and 1970s, was described as a method for exploring the qualitative and quantitative elements, patterns and structures of a problem under investigation (Van de Ven and Delbecq, 1972).

NGT seeks to generate and rank ideas, by encouraging contributions from a group or groups of participants, often from different disciplines or backgrounds, with varying perspectives on a problem, enabling input from those who prefer to think quietly and allowing discussion where there are areas of controversy or disagreement while avoiding this being dominated by one or a few individuals (Manera et al., 2019).

The original technique involves a series of phases: introduction, silent generation of ideas, round-robin listing of ideas on a flipchart, serial discussion of ideas, ranking or voting on ideas, feedback and discussion of ranking, re-ranking followed by a conclusion consisting of further feedback and a final discussion and summary.

The nominal or target group is a set of individuals who by virtue of their experience or expertise can offer insights into the problem being explored. The number of participants can vary, usually constituted in subgroups of around eight (the originators suggested five to nine) people, but multiple subgroups can enable a larger nominal group. The overall size can vary according to the relevant stakeholder groups which need to be involved and constraints imposed by the requirement to facilitate discussion in the meeting and resources needed such as time, space, travel costs or payment for contributors.

The 'facilitator', referred to also as the 'planner' by Van de Ven and Delbecq, needs to be skilled at facilitation and knowledgeable about the question under scrutiny. They introduce the meeting by clearly stating the aims and ground rules of the exercise at the outset, emphasising the need to focus on clarifying the problem before reaching solutions, stressing the importance of both objective and subjective perspectives on the topic and highlighting the value that each participant brings by virtue of their experience, views and knowledge of the problem under consideration (Van de Ven and Delbecq, 1972).

The silent generation of ideas in writing involves participants independently listing relevant ideas on the problem and possible solutions. The round-robin listing of ideas on a flipchart allows all the relevant ideas to be presented without judgment or discussion at this stage until sufficient ideas have been generated or no new ones are produced. The serial discussion involves presenting each of the ideas in turn for clarification, justification, debate, amalgamation, modification or addition of items. Ranking of the ideas takes place through independently and anonymously rating, ranking or voting in such a way that votes can be collated ready for feedback to participants. The feedback of ranking allows discussion as to whether and why participants agree with the priorities. This allows a further round of rating, feedback and discussion before the meeting concludes (Van de Ven and Delbecq, 1972).

There are various modifications of the technique, for example providing information to participants through written materials such as a literature review or survey beforehand; allowing small-group discussion before generation of ideas to stimulate thinking or allowing small groups to generate ideas collectively; using focus group methods for the small-group discussions; combining the round-robin listing and discussion phases (Manera et al., 2019); or conducting multiple NGT exercises with different stakeholder groups (Van de Ven and Delbecq, 1972). However, it is apparent that some of these modifications can be seen to conflict with the principles of the method as originally conceived.

Consensus Development Conference

The consensus development conference or panel was originated by the National Institutes of Health (NIH) in the USA during the 1970s for producing consensus statements that evaluated the benefits, costs, adverse effects and research gaps related to 'controversial medical interventions' or novel health technologies including drugs, devices and procedures (Wortman et al., 1988).

The original NIH process was loosely structured but fairly quickly developed into a more formalised process involving a group of around 10 to 15 selected experts, including a chairperson who helped form the consensus panel (Jacoby and Simopoulos, 1986). The panel met in a well-advertised public forum over a few days to address a consensus question. During the conference, they heard from various invited expert speakers who presented relevant evidence to them and answered questions from the panel and an audience of the public and medical professionals, who were also able to introduce new evidence, all of which informed deliberations between panel members leading to the production of a consensus statement for medical professionals and the public (Wortman et al., 1988).

An early process evaluation of the NIH process found problems with planning before, activities during and outputs and outcomes after NIH consensus conferences (Wortman et al., 1988). For example, before the conference there were problems with topic and question selection; bias in selecting panel members, chairs and speakers; lack of quality and comprehensiveness in prior evidence gathering, reviews and synthesis; and poor organisation of the process. During conferences, there were problems with managing disagreement and with insufficient time to draft consensus statements. Finally, post conference the variability in quality and accessibility of consensus statements, partly due to insufficient time to develop and draft them, and the failure to add anything new (Wortman et al., 1988) or to influence practice (Kosecoff et al., 1987), were raised as concerns.

This and other analyses led to recommendations for improving the process. Recommendations before the conference included greater transparency in topic and question selection, addressing wider issues such as costs, ethics and quality of life, being more open and transparent to engaging relevant expert representation when recruiting panel members, chairs and speakers (early conference members were only from a handful of US academic institutions) and providing more rigorous evidence synthesis and grading of quality of evidence to inform the panel. During the conference, more varied formats to engage debate and raise disagreements and more time to draft a clearer consensus statement, which also included areas where opinions differed, were advocated (Institute of Medicine, 1990; Wortman et al., 1988). Finally, post-conference recommendations were to provide a peer review of consensus statements (Jacoby, 1993) and to evaluate and develop the programme (Institute of Medicine, 1990).

The method has been developed or adapted since then by governments, national and international organisations, societies and committees to develop consensus guidelines and statements on a variety of health conditions and technologies, with the first UK consensus conference held in 1994 on coronary bypass grafting (Goodman and Baratz, 1990). The National Institute for Health and Care Excellence in the UK uses well-developed and -described processes for health technology appraisal, guidance development and related products such as best evidence summaries, pathways, standards and indicators (NICE, 2013), which are currently undergoing public consultation for further improvement.

Comparing Consensus Methods

When comparing these three methods, it is useful to compare and contrast the similarities and differences in their aims, structures, activities and intended outputs and outcomes.

As the name implies, they all seek to achieve consensus, where this is possible, but seek to achieve this in different ways and for slightly different purposes. Consensus conferences usually seek opinions on novel or mainstream health technologies or procedures to reach agreement on effectiveness, safety and other aspects of the intervention to guide healthcare practice and future research. The NGT is also designed to generate ideas as well as opinions on novel areas or topics. The Delphi process can generate new information but is better suited to prioritising areas of interest, such as future research areas or clinical indicators.

All three methods require skilled planning and organisation to maintain the engagement and input of participants in the process. The NGT also requires skilled facilitation, and consensus conferences need expert chairs to enable differences of opinion to be raised, aired and documented, whereas the Delphi exercise in its original form maintains the anonymity of participants.

Participants should reflect the diversity of stakeholder opinion needed to achieve valid judgments, and the method by which participants are selected will be a key factor in ensuring the validity and credibility of any consensus method. Participants should be selected through an open, transparent process, should represent their profession or stakeholder group, should include public and patient contributors (Waggoner et al., 2016) and should not have vested or conflicting interests (or these should be declared).

The number of participants will vary depending on the number of stakeholder groups who need to contribute, the range of expertise required and the resources and time available. Increasing numbers improve reliability and, to some extent, validity, while also increasing resource requirements of time and costs and risking greater disagreement and debating redundant or spurious information, which will require better facilitation and organisation. The minimum and ideal numbers vary from publication to publication but are said to be 10–15 for consensus conferences, 5–9 for nominal groups and 6–11 for the Delphi process (Waggoner et al., 2016). Multiples of these numbers are needed if there are multiple stakeholder groups, although the processes can become unmanageable with large numbers.

Information and cues are also important to inform the different approaches. Consensus panels should be provided in advance, with syntheses of quantitative and qualitative data in accessible formats (Murphy et al., 1998) and information from expert speakers to inform participants' judgments (Wortman et al., 1988). Nominal groups and Delphi panels also need to be provided with relevant information (Waggoner et al., 2016) upon which to base their opinions depending on the subject under discussion and what empirical data or information cues are available or appropriate.

The consensus conference usually makes group decisions during one or more meetings, whereas the NGT relies on two rounds of rating (sometimes more) and the Delphi process on at least two and usually three or four rounds to reach consensus. Rating, ranking or voting in the Delphi or NGT requires statistical analysis, feedback of individual and average (median) ratings and re-rating to achieve consensus.

All consensus exercises require dissemination and evaluation to encourage and determine the extent of implementation or uptake of the recommendations.

Examples of Consensus Studies

An early and influential example of a prehospital Delphi study was Snooks' study of prehospital research priorities (**Box 8.1**), which used a three-round Delphi (Snooks et al., 2009). Many of these priorities were investigated over the following decade, for

Box 8.1 Delphi Study Investigating Highest Prehospital Research Priorities (Snooks et al., 2009)

Snooks and colleagues used a Delphi process to identify the highest priorities for prehospital research in 2007–2008. The Delphi study was informed by a review of literature, policy documents and discussion between delegates at a national prehospital conference.

The Delphi process consisted of three rounds. The first round invited participants to comment on a grouped list of gaps previously identified and to suggest any missing topics. In the second round, participants were asked to prioritise each topic area, scoring from 1 (not important) to 9 (very important), allowing comments and research methods for each. In the third and final round, participants were provided with feedback in the form of group mean scores and comments from round two, and invited to adjust their own scores and suggest research methods after considering the views of others. Results from the final round were summarised to identify prehospital research priorities.

Overall, from 158 people from 10 organisations invited to participate, 40 people participated in the first round and 30 in rounds two and three.

The top ten priorities identified were:

1. Development of Emergency Medical Services (EMS) performance measures other than response times for use in performance management, audit and research

2. Prehospital clinical management of stroke

3. Safety, costs and benefits of alternatives to conveyance to hospital

4. Development of patient-focused clinical outcome measures

5. Methods for combining information on prehospital care and patient outcomes across ambulance service and other healthcare organisations

6. Developing interventions to appropriately manage the increase in 999 calls

7. Evaluation of mechanical aids for cardiopulmonary resuscitation

8. Nasal route for administration of pain relief

9. Alternatives to ambulance response or transport to emergency departments (EDs) for stroke

10. Clinical prehospital management of confused/aggressive patients with head injuries.

example performance (1) and outcome (5) measures (Siriwardena et al., 2010; Turner et al., 2019), safety of alternatives to conveyance (Coster et al., 2018b; O'Cathain et al., 2018), mechanical resuscitation aids (Perkins et al., 2015) and stroke care (Bath and Investigators, 2019; Price et al., 2020).

The Prehospital Outcomes for Evidence Based Evaluation (PhOEBE) programme (Turner et al., 2019), developed as a result of the previous prioritisation exercise, involved a nominal group and Delphi study (Coster et al., 2018a) (**Box 8.2**).

Box 8.2 The Prehospital Outcomes for Evidence Based Evaluation (PhOEBE) Programme (Turner et al., 2019)

The PhOEBE programme employed a three-stage consensus process of a modified nominal group, modified Delphi study and patient and public consensus workshop, to identify new ways of measuring ambulance service quality and performance incorporating service provider and public perspectives. The consensus processes involved representatives from ambulance services, patient and public contributors, academics, commissioners and policy makers.

A one-day nominal group event was attended by 42 (67%) of the 63 people who expressed an interest. Participants were separated in tables of six to eight participants facilitated by members of the research team, mixing different disciplines and public contributors. After introducing the aim and process for the day, candidate measures from **systematic reviews** were used as a starting point for group discussions. Facilitated small-group discussions were held for each group of measures where members were encouraged to add measures. The round-robin format ensured that each participant had an opportunity to contribute. Electronic voting was used to rank the importance of each measure or principle as a potential measure of good-quality ambulance service care. Nine measures were highly prioritised by more than three-quarters of consensus event participants, including measures relating to pain, patient experience, accuracy of dispatch decisions and patient safety (Coster et al., 2018a).

Twenty experts took part in a two-round Delphi process which was used to refine and prioritise the measures identified in the previous nominal group. Twenty measures in three domains scored highly (at least eight out of nine), indicating good consensus. Measures prioritised after two rounds included the proportion of calls correctly prioritised, time to definitive care and measures related to pain.

A consensus workshop including research presentations, facilitated discussions and electronic voting enabled 18 patient and public contributors to identify which measures they considered most important. Six were prioritised, including time to definitive care, response time, reduction in pain scores, calls correctly prioritised to appropriate levels of response and survival to hospital discharge for treatable emergency conditions (Irving et al., 2018).

The measures were developed to assess prehospital quality or performance over time, with most using routinely available data.

Summary

Consensus methods are helpful when a research question needs groups to reach agreement on policy or decision making in an area of uncertainty. The main consensus designs – Delphi process, NGT and consensus development conference – all have particular uses, advantages and disadvantages in exploring areas of uncertainty and prioritising areas for further practice, study or evaluation.

Further Reading

Jones, J. and Hunter, D. 1995. Consensus methods for medical and health services research. *BMJ*, 311, 376–380.

Rand corporation articles on the Delphi method: https://www.rand.org/topics/delphi-method.html.

References

Bath, P. M. and RIGHT-2 Investigators. 2019. Prehospital transdermal glyceryl trinitrate in patients with ultra-acute presumed stroke (RIGHT-2): An ambulance-based, randomised, sham-controlled, blinded, phase 3 trial. *Lancet*, 393, 1009–1020.

Bolger, F. and Wright, G. 2011. Improving the Delphi process: Lessons from social psychological research. *Technological Forecasting and Social Change*, 78, 1500–1513.

Bowling, A. 2009. *Research Methods in Health: Investigating Health and Health Services*. Maidenhead, Open University Press.

Brown, B. B. 1968. *Delphi Process: A Methodology Used for the Elicitation of Opinions of Experts*. Santa Monica, The Rand Corporation.

Coster, J. E. et al. 2018a. Prioritizing novel and existing ambulance performance measures through expert and lay consensus: A three-stage multimethod consensus study. *Health Expect*, 21, 249–260.

Coster, J. et al. 2018b. Outcomes for patients who contact the emergency ambulance service and are not transported to the emergency department: A data linkage study. *Prehospital Emergency Care*, 1–27.

Dalkey, N. 1967. Delphi. *Second Symposium on Long Range Forecasting and Planning*. Almagordo, New Mexico; RAND Corporation, Santa Monica.

Diamond, I. R. et al. 2014. Defining consensus: A systematic review recommends methodologic criteria for reporting of Delphi studies. *Journal of Clinical Epidemiology*, 67, 401–409.

Fink, A. et al. 1984. Consensus methods: Characteristics and guidelines for use. *American Journal of Public Health*, 74, 979–983.

Goodman, C. and Baratz, S. R. 1990. *Improving Consensus Development for Health Technology Assessment: An International Perspective*. National Academy Press, Washington DC.

Gugiu, M. R. et al. 2021. Development and validation of content domains for paramedic prehospital performance assessment: A focus group and delphi method approach. *Prehospital Emergency Care*, 25, 196–204.

Humphrey-Murto, S., Wood, T. J. and Varpio, L. 2017. When I say ... consensus group methods. *Medical Education*, 51, 994–995.

Irving, A. et al. 2018. A coproduced patient and public event: An approach to developing and prioritizing ambulance performance measures. *Health Expect*, 21, 230–238.

Jacoby, I. 1993. Consensus development at NIH: What went wrong. *Risk: Issues in Health and Safety*, 4, 133–142.

Jacoby, I. and Simopoulos, A. P. 1986. NIH consensus conferences: Guidelines and goals. *Journal of Nutrition*, 116, 312–316.

Jones, J. and Hunter, D. 1995. Consensus methods for medical and health services research. *BMJ*, 311, 376–380.

Kilner, T. 2004. Desirable attributes of the ambulance technician, paramedic, and clinical supervisor: Findings from a Delphi study. *Emergency Medicine Journal*, 21, 374–378.

Kosecoff, J. et al. 1987. Effects of the National Institutes of Health consensus development program on physician practice. *JAMA*, 258, 2708–2713.

Manera, K. et al. 2019. Consensus methods: Nominal group technique. *In:* Liamputtong, P. (Ed.) *Handbook of Research Methods in Health Social Sciences*. Singapore: Springer.

Morgan, M. G. 2014. Use (and abuse) of expert elicitation in support of decision making for public policy. *Proceedings of the National Academy of Sciences of the United States of America*, 111, 7176–7184.

Murphy, M. K. et al. 1998. Consensus development methods, and their use in clinical guideline development. *Health Technology Assessment*, 2, i–iv, 1–88.

Nice. 2013. *Guide to the Methods of Technology Appraisal 2013*, London, National Institute for Health and Care Excellence.

O'Cathain, A. et al. 2018. Understanding variation in ambulance service non-conveyance rates: A mixed methods study. *Health Services and Delivery Research*, 6, 1–191.

Perkins, G. D. et al. 2015. Mechanical versus manual chest compression for out-of-hospital cardiac arrest (PARAMEDIC): A pragmatic, cluster randomised controlled trial. *Lancet*, 385, 947–955.

Price, C. I. et al. 2020. Effect of an enhanced paramedic acute stroke treatment assessment on thrombolysis delivery during emergency stroke care: A cluster randomized clinical trial. *JAMA Neurology*, 77, 840–848.

Siriwardena, A. N. et al. 2010. Development and pilot of clinical performance indicators for English ambulance services. *Emergency Medicine Journal*, 27, 327–331.

Skrabanek, P. 1990. Nonsensus consensus. *Lancet*, 335, 1446–1447.

Snooks, H. et al. 2009. What are the highest priorities for research in emergency prehospital care? *Emergency Medicine Journal*, 26, 549–550.

Institute of Medicine. 1990. *Consensus Development at the NIH: Improving the Program: Report of a Study*, Washington, National Academy Press.

Turner, J. et al. 2019. Developing new ways of measuring the quality and impact of ambulance service care: The PhOEBE mixed-methods research programme. *Programme Grants for Applied Research*, 7, 1–90.

Van De Ven, A. H. and Delbecq, A. L. 1972. The nominal group as a research instrument for exploratory health studies. *American Journal of Public Health*, 62, 337–342.

Waggoner, J., Carline, J. D. and Durning, S. J. 2016. Is there a consensus on consensus methodology? Descriptions and recommendations for future consensus research. *Acadademic Medicine*, 91, 663–668.

Wortman, P. M., Vinokur, A. and Sechrest, L. 1988. Do consensus conferences work? A process evaluation of the NIH consensus development program. *Journal of Health Politics, Policy and Law*, 13, 469–498.

Chapter 9

Critically Appraising a Paper and Preparing a Paper for Publication

Bill Lord

Chapter Objectives

This chapter will cover:

- Rationale for the development of information literacy and critical appraisal skills
- Application of critical appraisal of the literature to clinical practice
- Finding information to answer a clinical or operational question
- Interpretation of research findings
- Identification of bias that may affect reliability of the data
- Preparing a paper for publication

Introduction

A healthcare colleague has discovered the following advice from a prominent person that recommends combination drug therapy – hydroxychloroquine and azithromycin – as an effective treatment for COVID-19 (Trump, 2020); see **Figure 9.1**.

Your colleague asks for your advice regarding the accuracy of this recommendation, as they have had clients enquiring about these drugs to treat COVID-19 symptoms. Hydroxychloroquine has been used for many years for malaria prophylaxis and for the treatment of rheumatoid arthritis and lupus. Azithromycin is a broad-spectrum macrolide antibiotic. As you are unaware of any clinical guidelines that recommend this combination therapy for the treatment of COVID-19 symptoms, you will need to critique the evidence for the use of these drugs for this purpose in order to provide correct advice to your colleague, as it is possible that the recommendation cited above may be incorrect, even though the author appears to have cited a biomedical journal within their Tweet to support their claim.

The Importance of Critical Evaluation of Information

Healthcare professionals have an obligation to maintain knowledge of contemporary evidence that underpins their practice so that patients receive appropriate, safe and

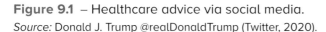

Mar 22, 2020

HYDROXYCHLOROQUINE & AZITHROMYCIN, taken together, have a real chance to be one of the biggest game changers in the history of medicine. The FDS has moved mountains – Thank You! Hopefully they will BOTH (H works better with A, International Journal of Antimicrobial Agents).....

....be put in use IMMEDIATELY. PEOPLE ARE DYING, MOVE FAST, and GOD BLESS EVERYONE!
@US_FDS @SteveFDS @CDCgov @DHSgov

@realDonaldTrump, Twitter, 12.13 AM . Mar 22, 2020

Figure 9.1 – Healthcare advice via social media.
Source: Donald J. Trump @realDonaldTrump (Twitter, 2020).

effective care. They also have an obligation to provide accurate heath advice to patients. This professional responsibility depends on the individual's ability to locate, analyse, evaluate and synthesise information that informs practice.

Guidelines supporting clinical practice should be supported by appropriate evidence. However, this has not always been possible due to the paucity of high-quality evidence informing paramedicine and emergency medicine. For example, paramedics in several countries routinely administered intravenous lidocaine bolus and infusions for ventricular ectopics in the presence of suspected myocardial infarction during the 1980s and 1990s, as it was believed that the presence of ectopic complexes increased the risk of ventricular tachycardia or fibrillation, particularly if an ectopic occurred during the relative refractory period of repolarisation (R-on-T phenomenon). Expert advice at the time was that lidocaine 'is of undoubted value in the treatment of ventricular extrasystoles' (Vincent, 1997). This was despite earlier evidence from prospective studies that found an increased mortality and increased risk of dysrhythmias such as atrioventricular block due to the pro-arrhythmic properties of the drug (Hine et al., 1989).

Early therapeutic recommendations were often based on low-quality evidence, or expert opinion in the absence of reliable evidence. While recommendations were usually made in good faith based on a mechanistic view of pharmacology and human physiology, many recommendations were modified following the publication of high-level (**randomised controlled trials** or **systematic reviews** of randomised controlled trials) evidence that challenged these assumptions or opinions.

Much of the evidence that supports current practice is generated from research that uses appropriate research methods to answer questions presented as a hypothesis or as **outcomes** of interest. This process of scientific enquiry needs to be rigorous and transparent to ensure that recommendations can be safely applied to the care of patients. Rigour arises from the process of conducting the research, which usually involves ethical considerations before a study is approved, the methods used to conduct the research and the peer-review process that acts as a check before the results are published. However, not all research that has been through a peer-review process is free from **bias** or error, and it is important to know how to undertake a critique of the literature before assuming that the recommendations are fit for purpose.

In addition, there are many other sources of health information that can be accessed by both patients and healthcare professionals, and it is important that this information is subject to a screening process to assess **reliability**. The growth of social media can have positive benefits in enabling rapid communication of important data. However, this form of media has also enabled the spread of misinformation and conspiracy theories, which has forced public health organisations such as the World Health Organisation to focus on 'myth busting' associated with the rapid rise of social media misinformation (Nguyen and Catalan, 2020).

The rapid growth of dubious sources of health information during the COVID-19 pandemic is a good example of the need to assess the basis for recommendations that may pose a risk to public safety. Examples include therapy for treatment and prophylaxis of viral infections and recommendations regarding infection prevention that have no scientific basis, or that include claims that are counter to established public health strategies. In the case of hydroxychloroquine, research trials were rapidly established due to high-level political endorsements that could have increased the risk of adverse outcomes if followed by members of the public. Yet in a race to publish data that might inform health decisions, *The Lancet*, a long-established medical journal, published a study of the effectiveness of hydroxychloroquine that was soon retracted due to concerns regarding the accuracy or even the existence of the data used to undertake the analysis (Mehra et al., 2020). Investigations revealed that the hospitals that were cited as having provided patient data for the analysis denied having participated in the study. The study design in this case was a retrospective observation of previously obtained patient heath data. This type of study is prone to errors due to having no control over the quality of the data included in the analysis. The more robust type of study design to answer a therapeutic efficacy and safety study is a randomised controlled study (see **Chapter 5: Experimental and Quasi-experimental Designs**).

This chapter provides a foundation for understanding the process of **critical appraisal** of information that may be used to inform your practice. There are many excellent sources for further information, including templates that can be used to appraise research based on the study design, for example, the checklists developed by the Critical Appraisal Skills Programme at the Oxford Centre for Triple Value

Healthcare (Critical Appraisal Skills Programme, 2020). These are licensed under a Creative Commons Licence, making them freely available for non-commercial use. For qualitative research, there are also reliable templates used to evaluate the study design and the outcomes (Lockwood et al., 2015). As such, this chapter does not aim to provide a comprehensive compendium to critiquing the evidence, but rather an introduction to guide further study.

Using Evidence to Inform Practice

Your health service is considering the addition of a new inhalational analgesic to the formulary for the treatment of acute pain. The only data describing safety and efficacy consist of several **observational studies** that report good efficacy and few adverse effects. Large observational studies can provide useful information about therapeutic efficacy, but these studies should clearly outline the limitations of the data. An example is research published by Middleton and colleagues who reported efficacy of three analgesic agents used by paramedics in an Australian ambulance service (Middleton et al., 2010). In their study, the reported limitations included missing data in almost half the cases that were eligible for inclusion in the analysis, potential inaccuracies in the way that paramedics recorded the patient data and the inability to reliably record adverse drug effects.

To obtain more reliable data on drug efficacy and safety, higher levels of evidence such as randomised controlled trials (RCTs) are required, and these have only recently been published to enable a higher level of confidence about the use of one of these agents (Borobia et al., 2020). Nevertheless, there were also limitations in the RCT study due to the inability to blind clinicians to the treatment provided, and potential variations in the way that the 'standard treatment' arm was managed. In addition, the authors did not report statistical power calculations, meaning that the sample size may have been too small to reliably identify a difference in outcome. These examples show that all research is potentially associated with errors of design or analysis, or bias in reporting, and that the peer-review process is not always able to detect these problems. This begs the question 'how can I know what evidence is fit for purpose?'. This chapter aims to provide information to enable foundational skills in the critical appraisal of research outcomes.

How to Critique a Research Paper

You may encounter information from sources including your professional networks that appears to be relevant to your practice, or you might have a clinical or operational question that requires a focused search for information to answer your question. When critiquing papers, the study design will determine the approach to analysing the research. Templates are available to assist with this process (Critical Appraisal Skills Programme, 2020). For this section of the chapter, we are going to critique papers that describe the effectiveness of a therapeutic device, and then later look at how to frame a question, and to search for and locate information that addresses a question you have developed. This will describe an approach to critiquing the methodological quality of the paper to assess the validity, reliability and applicability of these data.

The steps involved in locating information relating to a clinical question are as follows:

- Frame a question that will guide your search using a format such as **PICO** (Population, Intervention, Comparator, Outcome).

- Undertake multiple database searches using appropriate search terms.

- Limit the results to those that meet your inclusion/exclusion criteria. Exclusions may include age, study design or those studies undertaken on animals.

When you have located the papers that address your question, undertake the following checks:

- Did the authors describe their hypothesis or outcomes of interest?

- Did the authors use an appropriate study design and statistical analysis? For example, studies describing therapies require experimental methods such as blinded RCTs (while acknowledging that it is impossible to blind all types of intervention to the study participants; for example, when comparing standard cardiopulmonary resuscitation (CPR) outcomes with CPR using a mechanical chest compression device, it is very difficult to conceal the active arm of the study). For research that seeks to understand the participants' lived experience of a phenomenon of interest, several qualitative methods may be used.

- What is the 'level of evidence'?

- Is there evidence of bias?

- Do the results demonstrate an outcome that is statistically significant? Are the results clinically significant?

Critiquing Research Papers: A Case Study

You are working in an area of your organisation that has responsibility for clinical standards and **quality improvement**. Your manager has recently attended a conference where she has learnt about a new airway device that is promoted as improving outcomes from cardiac arrest. The manager has brought you a sample of the device as well as marketing brochures that cite evidence used to support the claim for improvements in patient survival and asks you whether this device should be added to the management of cardiac arrest across the organisation.

The device is known as an impedance threshold device (ITD) and the marketing material includes claims that the device improves perfusion during CPR by changing intrathoracic pressure to increase preload and improve cerebral perfusion by reducing intracranial pressure. Your task is to review the literature relating to the efficacy of this device to make a recommendation regarding implementation in your practice setting. It should be noted that this is not a critique of the device or the vendor, but rather a critique of the literature that describes trials of this device.

You note that the marketing brochure for this device claims that when used in conjunction with high-quality CPR, survival can be improved by 25% or more. Citations in support of this claim include the following:

> Yannopoulos, D. et al. 2015. Quality of CPR: An important effect modifier in cardiac arrest clinical outcomes and intervention effectiveness trials. *Resuscitation*, 94, 106–113.

When you source the full text of this paper, you note that this is a post hoc analysis of data from a previously published study. The primary study was:

> Aufderheide, T. P. et al. 2011. A trial of an impedance threshold device in out-of-hospital cardiac arrest. *The New England Journal of Medicine*, 365, 798–806.

These papers will be analysed in chronological order using the previous checklist.

Did the Authors Describe Their Hypothesis or Outcomes of Interest?

Aufderheide et al. (2011) aimed to compare the use of an active ITD with that of a sham ITD in adult patients with a diagnosis of non-traumatic out-of-hospital cardiac arrest where Emergency Medical Services (EMS) provided CPR across ten locations in the USA and Canada.

Rather than stating a null hypothesis, the authors describe a primary outcome of interest as survival to hospital discharge with satisfactory neurological function considered to be a score of ≤3 on the modified Rankin Scale (mRS). Secondary outcomes of interest were return of spontaneous circulation (ROSC) on arrival at the emergency department, survival to hospital admission and survival to hospital discharge.

Did the Authors Use Appropriate Study Design and Statistical Analysis?

The study undertaken by Aufderheide and colleagues (2011) was a large multicentre clinical trial involving adult patients who were randomly assigned to have either an active ITD or a sham device included as part of their CPR treatment. A power calculation was reported by Aufderheide et al. (2011) to determine the sample size that needed to be recruited to minimise the possibility of a chance outcome rather than actual effect. Each device was packaged in a way that blinded the participants to the device (active or sham). Each was identified for analysis by means of a numerical code known only to the data coordinators.

Cases where the study conduct deviated from the **protocol** should be excluded from analysis, but the occurrence of protocol deviation cannot be determined from the information in the paper.

The z-statistic was used to compare outcomes between the two groups for the primary outcome. A z-value allows calculation of the probability of difference in proportions or means between two groups if the groups have normal distributions. Differences between each group in rates of survival to discharge with satisfactory functional status were also estimated with the use of a multiple linear regression that was adjusted for baseline characteristics. The study design and the statistical analysis were appropriate for the study type and outcomes of interest.

What Was the 'Level of Evidence'?

An RCT is an appropriate design for research that investigates a therapeutic intervention.

Is There Evidence of Bias?

Bias may be difficult to ascertain but the concept should be understood, as bias can affect the validity and reliability of research results. Problems that lead to bias include errors in the design, implementation, data analysis or reporting. For example, the blinding of participants to the intervention (active or sham) reduces bias that may occur in an unblinded study, where knowledge of the treatment may influence the care provided and therefore the study outcomes. The Cochrane Collaboration has developed tools for assessing bias in randomised trials, and this should be consulted for additional detail (Higgins et al., 2011).

Do the Results Demonstrate an Outcome That Is Statistically Significant? Are the Results Clinically Significant?

The study included 8,718 patients in the analysis, with 260 patients (6.0%) in the sham-ITD group and 254 patients (5.8%) in the active-ITD group meeting the primary outcome – survival to hospital discharge with a mRS score of ≤3. The 95% **confidence interval** (CI) was reported to be −1.1 to 0.8, and the $P = 0.71$.

To effectively critique research outcomes, you must be able to interpret CIs and P values. The difference between groups in this study was considered significant if the P value was less than 0.05, as this indicates strong evidence against a null hypothesis (null being no difference between the groups), meaning that the hypothesis can be rejected. In this case the P value is greater than 0.05, meaning that the null hypothesis cannot be rejected. The figure used for the level of significance in this case (0.05) infers a 1 in 20 chance that the result is wrong, or that it may have occurred through chance.

However, as the P value provides limited information about the difference between sample groups, it is common for a CI to also be reported. The CI is used to compare the means of two or more groups, in this case treatment arms of the study. The CI shows the magnitude of the plausible range of difference between groups for the true population, which helps with the interpretation of the statistical significance and the clinical significance of a treatment. The CI reported in this case indicates a 95% chance that the indicated range bounded by the upper and lower limits contains the true population difference in survival to hospital discharge. Because this is a two-sided outcome (survival can be better or worse comparing sham with active device), a CI must not include zero, as this would indicate no difference in the outcome of interest in the groups being studied. In this case the CI ranges from −1.1 to 0.8, meaning that there is no difference in the odds of survival between groups (some did better, some did worse). The authors therefore concluded that 'use of the active ITD did not significantly improve survival with satisfactory function' (Aufderheide et al., 2011).

When the CI is used to measure intervention effect (which may be reported as an odds ratio, hazard ratio or risk ratio), this typically involves a log transformation and may be reported as a log odds ratio. When ratio statistics are reported, the lowest possible value is zero, the number 1 indicates no intervention effect and the highest possible value is infinity. Therefore, you will see discussion of the CI 'crossing one' in relation to no treatment effect. For example, a paper that aimed to investigate the effect of patient and paramedic gender on analgesic interventions reported the odds ratio of analgesic administration by paramedic gender, using female gender as the reference (odds 1.0). This showed that the odds ratio (95% CI) for male paramedic administration of analgesia was 0.97 (0.89–1.06). As the CI crossed 1.0 there was no treatment difference, which is also confirmed by a P value of 0.47. However, the results showed that male patients (compared with female patients) had greater odds of receiving paramedic-initiated analgesia with a 95% CI of 1.58 (1.49–1.68). This can be interpreted to mean that male patients were on average 58% more likely to receive analgesia than female patients (P < 0.0001) (Lord et al., 2014).

This final section of the checklist also asks whether the result is *clinically significant*. It is common to see results reported as statistically significant when the difference raises concerns about whether this is associated with clinical benefit or a clear clinical difference. For example, in a study that investigated the correlation between patient vital signs and pain severity score in the paramedic practice setting, the authors found no statistically significant difference between pulse rate or systolic blood pressure and patient pain severity score. There was a statistically significant association between respiratory rate and pain severity, with each one-point increase in pain severity on a 0–10 pain score associated with an increase in respiratory rate of 0.16 breaths per minute. However, the authors were probably correct in concluding that 'the degree of change was so small it cannot be considered to be clinically significant' (Lord and Woollard, 2011).

Can This Device Be Recommended for Your Practice?

Based on the outcomes of the Aufderheide study, it may be difficult to convince senior managers that this device should be implemented in your practice. However, a post hoc analysis of the data from the Aufderheide study was undertaken by Yannopoulos and colleagues, in which the authors studied the interaction of *quality of the CPR* and the use of an ITD, and it is the latter study that is listed on the product information to support a claim of increased survival from cardiac arrest (Yannopoulos et al., 2015).

The dataset from Aufderheide et al.'s (2011) prospective study included CPR parameters captured by thoracic impedance recorded from defibrillation electrodes or from an accelerometer placed on the patient's chest. The captured data included chest compression rate, compression depth and fraction.

The paper by Yannopoulos and colleagues (2015) (**Box 9.1**) was undertaken to determine whether the quality of CPR was an outcome modifier in the earlier study undertaken by Aufderheide et al. (2011). The authors listed the primary endpoint of the study as the 'interaction between the three individual components used to assess the quality of CPR provided (rate, depth and fraction) and their combinations, the intervention (sham or active ITD); and survival to hospital discharge with mRS ≤ 3' (Yannopoulos et al., 2015).

Yannopoulos et al. found that when 'acceptable' quality CPR was performed, use of the active ITD increased survival to hospital discharge with modified Rankin Scale score ≤ 3 compared to the sham device (61/848 [7.2%] versus 34/827 [4.1%], respectively; p = 0.006) (Yannopoulos et al., 2015). However, as CPR quality was not a component of the initial research question or hypothesis, there were considerable missing data in the subsequent post hoc analysis, with compression depth data available for only 43% of subjects (Yannopoulos et al., 2015). In addition, the authors reported that when CPR was performed outside the range of acceptable values, the addition of an active ITD significantly decreased the rate of survival to hospital discharge with mRS score ≤ 3 compared to the sham ITD (34/1013 (3.4%) for the active ITD versus 62/1061 (5.8%) for the sham ITD, p = 0.0071) (Yannopoulos et al., 2015).

Is the outcome of this analysis sufficient for you to recommend the introduction of the ITD to your practice setting? What may some of the **confounders** be in this later study?

Post hoc analysis refers to an investigation that occurs after a study has been conducted. There are increased risks of bias when undertaking post hoc analysis that attempts to fit a hypothesis to an observed result. There is a risk that researchers have undertaken post hoc analysis to test data in a way that fits a favourable result. This is known as confirmation bias, and this also occurs when people source information that aims to confirm their existing beliefs.

This does not necessarily negate the result, as this type of analysis can identify patterns that may be used to inform further research that sets out to test the new hypothesis using appropriate experimental designs. However, as Olasveengen and colleagues remind us in their editorial regarding this research, 'science needs to be based on *a priori* tested hypothesis, not post hoc analysis', and the results 'are not actionable and should not guide current practice' (Olasveengen et al., 2015).

> ### Box 9.1 Critical Analysis Exercise
>
> Locate the Yannopoulos study (2015) and critique this paper using the following checklist:
> - Did the authors describe their hypothesis or outcomes of interest?
> - Did the authors use appropriate study design and statistical analysis?
> - What is the 'level of evidence'?
> - Is there evidence of bias?
> - Do the results demonstrate an outcome that is statistically significant? Are the results clinically significant?

Table 9.1 – PICO question.

Population	Who are the relevant patients or the target audience, or what is the condition or disease of interest?
Intervention	What intervention is being considered?
Comparator	What is the main comparator or alternative to the intervention that you want to assess?
Outcomes	What are the main outcomes of interest?

To determine whether the ITD should be considered for implementation in your organisation, further evidence needs to be located and critiqued. The next step involves searching for evidence based on your data question.

Finding Evidence Based on a PICO Question

A search for evidence relating to a question regarding a clinical intervention such as the effectiveness of the ITD requires the use of a PICO question (Richardson et al., 1995); see **Table 9.1**.

When addressing a question that relies on qualitative data, the PICO is often modified to read Population or Problem, Interest and Context in which the study is set (see **Chapter 1: Introduction, Figure 1.5**).

P – Adults with a non-traumatic out-of-hospital cardiac arrest treated by paramedics

I – Cardiopulmonary resuscitation (CPR) where an impedance threshold device was used

C – Standard (CPR) using a sham device

O – Survival to discharge.

Conducting a comprehensive search for evidence that addresses your research question is a complex task and you should ideally seek specialist advice, such as a librarian responsible for your field of study at an academic library. Academic libraries offer access to several databases to enable searches for relevant research, and these can usually simultaneously search multiple databases. Access may also be available through organisations such as the National Institute for Health and Care Excellence (NICE) in the UK, with the organisation providing the Healthcare Databases Advanced Search (NICE, 2020). Staff working for health services, including ambulance services, may find that they have access to resources through the Library and Knowledge Service for NHS Ambulance Services in England (Library and Knowledge Service for NHS Ambulance Services in England, 2020).

In this case, we will search for evidence and then filter the results to find the highest level of evidence that answers your research question – a systematic review of RCTs. The reason for limiting the search to systematic reviews is that this type of research is one that synthesises results from other homogenous RCTs, and as such this represents appropriate and high-level evidence for assessing studies that address the safety and efficacy of therapies (see **Chapter 1: Introduction, Figure 1.1** for **hierarchy of evidence**, and **Chapter 3: Systematic Reviews** for further discussion of systematic reviews). For additional information about the different levels of evidence and application based on type of study, see the Oxford Centre for Evidence-Based Medicine (Howick et al., 2009). To enable effective searching for research pertaining to paramedicine or out-of-hospital care, the search filter developed by Olaussen and colleagues is recommended (Olaussen et al., 2017).

The example of a search shown in **Figure 9.2** uses the MEDLINE database. This is a comprehensive biomedicine and life science database managed by the US National Library of Medicine that contains citations from over 5,200 journals. Other databases that you may need to consider include CINAHL, PsycINFO, Embase and the Cochrane Central Register of Controlled Trials (CENTRAL).

The results of this search show that two studies are systematic reviews of RCTs. One of these combines active compression-decompression resuscitation and an impedance threshold device, which confounds the findings as it is not clear which of these two interventions influenced the result (Wang et al., 2015). The other was published in 2008 and included five RCTs (Cabrini et al., 2008). This study found improvements in ROSC when the ITD was included in the management of cardiac arrest, but found no effect on favourable neurologic outcomes in survivors nor an improved survival at the longest available follow-up (Cabrini et al., 2008).

Of the ten results that were limited to RCTs, only one meets the outcome inclusion criterion (survival to hospital discharge). This was the 2011 study previously discussed, which showed that 'the ITD did not significantly improve survival with satisfactory function among patients with out-of-hospital cardiac arrest' (Aufderheide et al., 2011).

▼ Search History (8)

# ▲	Searches	Results	Type	Actions
1	impedance threshold device. mp. [mp=title, abstract, original title, name of substance word, subject heading word, floating sub-heading word, keyword heading word, organism supplementary concept word, protocol supplementary concept word, rare disease supplementary concept word, unique identifier, synonyms]	111	Advanced	Display Results | More ▼
2	cardiac arrest.mp. [mp=title, abstract, original title, name of substance word, subject heading word, floating sub-heading word, keyword heading word, organism supplementary concept word, protocol supplementary concept word, rare disease supplementary concept word, unique identifier, synonyms]	31106	Advanced	Display Results | More ▼
3	cardiopulmonary resuscitation.mp. [mp=title, abstract, original title, name of substance word, subject heading word, floating sub-heading word, keyword heading word, organism supplementary concept word, protocal supplementary concept word, rare disease supplementary concept word, unique identifier, synonyms]	22707	Advanced	Display Results | More ▼
4	2 or 3	43700	Advanced	Display Results | More ▼
5	1 and 4	84	Advanced	Display Results | More ▼
6	limit 5 to (english language and humans)	48	Advanced	Display Results | More ▼
7	limit 6 to randomized controlled trial	10	Advanced	Display Results | More ▼
8	limit 5 to "systematic review"	2	Advanced	Display Results | More ▼

Figure 9.2 – Example of a search strategy.

Development of clinical practice guidelines is a complex process, and there are several systems currently used to appraise the strength and quality of the evidence that may inform guideline development. One that is widely used is the **Grading of Recommendations Assessment, Development and Evaluation (GRADE)** system for grading evidence (Guyatt et al., 2008b). Healthcare organisations that are responsible for developing clinical practice guidelines should use a rigorous and validated method of evaluating the evidence to inform guideline development and updates. Guidelines that inform resuscitation are published by the organisations that comprise the International Liaison Committee on Resuscitation. The UK member is the Resuscitation Council UK. The last major review of the evidence published in 2015 did not recommend the routine use of the ITD (Soar et al., 2015).

Levels of Evidence

There are several approaches used to rank the level of evidence. These typically place the following at the highest level of reliability: high-quality evidence arising from more than one RCT; **meta-analysis** of high-quality RCTs; and one or more RCTs corroborated by high-quality registry studies. Consensus of expert opinion is rated the lowest level of evidence (American Heart Association, 2019). However, the GRADE criteria use a simplified method, with quality adjusted based on assessment of bias, limited or imprecise data, study limitations or inconsistency in methods:

Randomised trial = high quality

Quasi-randomised trial = moderate quality

Observational study = low quality

Any other evidence = very low quality

(Guyatt et al., 2008a).

Problems Associated With Low Levels of Evidence

Clinical practice may be informed by evidence from observational studies and expert consensus opinion where higher levels of evidence are unavailable. However, the limitations of the data arising from these sources should be recognised. Other types of evidence such as case reports can inform practice by relating rare cases, diagnostic findings and adverse effects. When reading a case report, you should check that the patient demographics and history are reported, along with the clinical features of the case. Diagnostic tests should be appropriate and clearly described. Interventions and post-intervention changes in the patient's condition are important, but there is a risk that interventions may not be directly related to the observed clinical course. The following example reinforces this point.

Attributing Treatment and Effect: A Case Study

In 2020, a case report was published in the *Journal of Pediatric, Maternal and Family Health, Chiropractic* that reported on the 'Resolution of Abnormal Pulse Oximetry Measured in Real-Time in a Neonate with Vertebral Subluxation' (Osuna and Perez, 2020).

This report describes a home birth with a midwife in attendance. The report states that the midwife placed a pulse oximeter probe on the newborn's foot at three minutes after an uncomplicated delivery and noted a saturation reading of 73%. The APGAR score was noted to be 7/10 at one minute and four minutes post-delivery. The midwife is described to have administered oxygen, but the method is not documented. The oxygen saturation (SpO_2) was documented to be 93–95% following oxygen therapy, but there was still apparent concern that the baby was hypoxic. At this point a chiropractor (the author) provided the following treatment:

'After an in-depth consultation with the parents and the attending midwife, a pediatric chiropractor evaluated the newborn for the presence of vertebral subluxations. Special attention was placed on the upper cervical spine as it is a common area of trauma during the birth process. It is important to understand that even when pediatric cervical injuries in general are a rare occurrence, birth related neck trauma is many times unpublicized and therefore not treated accordingly'

(Osuna and Perez, 2020).

Oxygen saturation was reported to have improved following this manipulation. The conclusion states that 'this case study provides supporting evidence of the benefits of subluxation-based chiropractic care in the improvement of pulse oximetry readings in neonates' (Osuna and Perez, 2020).

Before you consider recommending chiropractic manipulation to manage presumed hypoxia in the newborn, you need to consider whether the treatment provided can be reliably associated with the observed outcome. Newborns normally have SpO_2 levels that are lower than the normal range in an infant, but the value gradually improves in the first few minutes following birth due to the normal transition from oxygenation provided by the placenta to foetal respiration and oxygenation. The APGAR of 7/10 represents a value that would be considered normal in a newborn, and pulse oximetry in this case did not appear to be indicated. The spinal manipulation may therefore be unrelated to the changes in oxygen saturation observed in an uncomplicated full-term birth, and as such the treatment and conclusion appear to be unwarranted. Although an extreme example, this highlights the importance of using high-level evidence to inform practice.

When assessing the reliability of data published in any journal, it is important to consider the credibility of the source, as there are increasing numbers of journals that do not meet standards such as the Committee on Publication Ethics' (COPE) Code of Conduct for Journal Publishers. Further information about 'predatory journals' is included in the following section.

Preparing a Paper for Publication

At some stage you may wish to write up the results of a literature review, scoping review or research project that you are undertaking. This may arise from a workplace project or be an outcome of a course of education that requires a research project. If you have done a lot of work to create new knowledge, this needs to be shared with your peers and others with an interest in your field of study. Much research is done to satisfy assessment requirements in a higher education programme of study but is never published. If good research is to inform and transform practice, it needs to be disseminated.

Where to Publish?

The choice of forums for the dissemination of your research depends on the intended audience and type of research. You should look at where similar types of research have been published and develop a shortlist, as you should know that journals receive many more manuscripts than they can reasonably publish, and as such you should prepare for some rejections. This sometimes occurs before your manuscript goes to peer review when the editor has assessed your submission and determined that it does not fit their aims or target audience.

You should also be aware that there are many unreputable and unethical journals that seek to publish manuscripts for a fee, often without a rigorous peer review. These are known as 'predatory journals', and they have had exponential growth in recent times. Databases such as Cabells Scholarly Analytics may be accessible through academic libraries to assist with selecting appropriate publication options and to identify predatory journals (Cabells, 2020).

Once you have a shortlist of potential publishers, it is important to ensure that you have read the 'information for authors' available on the website of your prospective publisher to reduce the risk of rejection. If you have research findings that have relevance to practitioners working in paramedicine or ambulance services, it may be wise to select potential publishers who specialise in this market. Remember that several high-quality emergency medicine journals will accept articles with a prehospital focus. For example, the *Emergency Medicine Journal* based in the UK will accept manuscripts that are likely to be of interest to physicians, nurses and paramedics. If you have undertaken qualitative research, you should aim for publication in journals that specialise in this form of research in your area of interest.

Some journals will be explicit in the types of studies they will not consider for publication. For example, advice to prospective authors published by *Advances in Health Sciences Education* outline several research methods that will not be considered, including reports of self-assessment of knowledge and skill development or self-assessed and reported confidence or competence in performance following an educational intervention (*Advances in Health Sciences Education*, n.d.).

Drafting Your Manuscript

You need to consider the style requirement for each journal on your shortlist. These will differ based on the type of research you are publishing, but there will be differences between journals in the same field of interest, for example, emergency medicine. You must ensure that you adhere to style requirements; otherwise, your manuscript may be rejected at an early stage of submission by the production team even before it reaches the editor. Style refers to the way in which your manuscript is structured, but there will also be spelling and referencing styles to consider. For example, publishers in North America will expect that spelling is consistent with local convention, which may mean dropping vowels (oedema versus edema). The easiest way to change the grammar is to select the local language in your word processor.

Because referencing styles may vary considerably between journals, the use of referencing software is highly recommended. Use one of the popular programmes to store references and insert these in your manuscript and ensure that the programme allows output styles to be quickly changed across the entire document. Do not be tempted to manually insert references, as this will cause considerable grief when you need to make global changes in your manuscript.

The typical layout of a manuscript that reports outcomes of observational or experimental studies includes these section headings:

- Introduction
- Methods
- Results
- Discussion
- Conclusion.

Subheadings can be included where needed and are again often a style requirement of some journals. In addition, an abstract is normally required and should be written when the first draft of the manuscript is complete to ensure that the content is consistent with the main manuscript. Ensure that you adhere to published word limits for the abstract and manuscript. You should try to find similar articles in the journal of choice to ensure that your style is consistent with previously published research. The exemplar used for these style recommendations is:

> Siriwardena, A. N. et al. 2019. Patient and clinician factors associated with prehospital pain treatment and outcomes: Cross sectional study. *American Journal of Emergency Medicine*, 37, 266–271.

Introduction

This is a critical component of your manuscript, as it 'sells' the research to the reader. You need to succinctly explain why this research has been undertaken, why it is important and how you are going to present the results. You should assume that the reader is not familiar with your specialisation of field or practice when you write this. Justification for the research should demonstrate a clear gap or unmet need and be supported by evidence that you have undertaken a literature search and critiqued the literature to identify a need for your research. The introduction should also include your hypothesis or research aims.

Methods

This section contains the details of population of interest or population sample, selection criteria, sample size, the statistical tests used to analyse the data and any ethical considerations. It needs to be clear that the statistical tests used were 'fit for purpose'. Information should include the data collected, outcomes of interest and the type of analysis undertaken. Subheadings may be used to differentiate sections, such as 'Study design and setting' and 'Data analysis'. Many journals now require the use of reporting guidelines that standardise the presentation of data. For example, **Strengthening the Reporting of OBservational Studies in Epidemiology (STROBE)** guidelines and checklists are available for reporting observational studies (von Elm et al., 2007). A list of the guidelines available for specific study designs is available from the **Enhancing the QUAlity** and **Transparency Of health Research (EQUATOR)** Network (see https://www .equator-network.org/).

Results

Outcomes of the data analysis are presented in this section. This normally includes an initial table that contains information about the study population such as age, sex and other relevant demographic information. A figure that shows the sample population and the effect on sample size after adding exclusion criteria such as missing data or patients lost to follow-up is also recommended. The results should reflect the investigations described in the Methods section and be presented in the same order. The primary outcome of interest should be reported in a table. Avoid duplicating data in the body of the manuscript where this is already described in a table. Comparative statistics such as the difference in means or odds ratios must include a 95% CI. P values are also typically reported; however, this information is somewhat redundant as significance can be derived from the CI. Avoid the temptation to discuss the results in this section; leave this for the following section.

Discussion

A summary of your results should then lead to a discussion of the implications for practice and a comparison of your results with previous research where applicable. The limitations of your research must be addressed, and this can be done here or in a separate section depending on the style requirements of the journal.

Conclusion

This provides an opportunity for a succinct drawing together of the results and for a discussion of 'where next?'. This is one section that readers may read first, so you need to ensure that it can stand alone and clearly convey the outcome of your study.

Finally, remember to acknowledge organisations that supported this research through access to data or in-kind support. Also acknowledge research assistants, proofreaders and statisticians if they do not appear on the list of authors.

Summary

Information relating to healthcare continues to grow rapidly, even though much of this is of questionable quality. Although it may be assumed that research published in peer-reviewed scientific journals is reliable and of high quality, data must be subjected to further scrutiny before it should be used to inform the community or to guide practice. Healthcare professionals have an obligation to maintain knowledge of contemporary evidence relating to their scope of practice, and this requires information literacy skills that include the ability to analyse, evaluate and synthesise information that informs safe and effective practice. This chapter provides the foundation skills required to underpin this important professional obligation. Advice regarding the preparation of your own publication is also provided. For those interested in more detailed information on critical appraisal, the following resources are recommended.

Further Reading

Bootland, D. et al. 2017. *Critical Appraisal from Papers to Patient: A Practical Guide*. Boca Raton, CRC Press.

Greenhalgh, T., 2019. *How to Read a Paper: The Basics of Evidence-based Medicine and Healthcare*, 6th Edn. Newark, John Wiley and Sons.

References

Advances in Health Sciences Education. n.d. Aims and scope. Available at: https://www.springer .com/journal/10459/aims-and-scope [Accessed 18 November 2020].

American Heart Association. 2019. Applying class of recommendations and level of evidence to clinical strategies, interventions, treatments, or diagnostic testing in patient care. Dallas: AHA. Available at: https://cpr.heart.org/en/resuscitation-science/cpr-and-ecc-guidelines/tables/ applying-class-of-recommendation-and-level-of-evidence [Accessed 12 December 2020].

Aufderheide, T. P. et al. 2011. A trial of an impedance threshold device in out-of-hospital cardiac arrest. *The New England Journal of Medicine*, 365, 798–806.

Borobia, A. M. et al. 2020. Inhaled methoxyflurane provides greater analgesia and faster onset of action versus standard analgesia in patients with trauma pain: Inmediate: A randomized controlled trial in emergency departments. *Annals of Emergency Medicine*, 75, 315–328.

Cabells. 2020. Scholarly analytics, journalytics. Available at: https://www2.cabells.com/about-journalytics [Accessed 15 November 2021].

Cabrini, L. et al. 2008. Impact of impedance threshold devices on cardiopulmonary resuscitation: A systematic review and meta-analysis of randomized controlled studies. *Critical Care Medicine*, 36, 1625–1632.

Critical Appraisal Skills Programme. 2020. CASP checklists. Oxford, CASP. Available at: https:// casp-uk.net/casp-tools-checklists/ [Accessed 12 December 2020].

Guyatt, G. H. et al. 2008a. What is "quality of evidence" and why is it important to clinicians? *BMJ*, 336, 995–998.

Guyatt, G. H. et al. 2008b. Rating quality of evidence and strength of recommendations: GRADE: An emerging consensus on rating quality of evidence and strength of recommendations. *BMJ*, 336, 924–926.

Higgins, J. P. et al. 2011. The Cochrane Collaboration's tool for assessing risk of bias in randomised trials. *BMJ*, 343, D5928.

Hine, L. K. et al. 1989. Meta-analytic evidence against prophylactic use of lidocaine in acute myocardial infarction. *Archives of Internal Medicine*, 149, 2694–2698.

Howick, J. et al. 2009. *Oxford Centre for Evidence-Based Medicine: Levels of Evidence*. Oxford, University of Oxford, Centre for Evidence-Based Medicine.

Library and Knowledge Service for NHS Ambulance Services in England. 2020. Welcome to the library. Bolton: Health Education England (HEE) and the National Education Network for Ambulance Services (NENAS). Available at: https://ambulance.libguides.com/home1/home [Accessed 12 December 2020].

Lockwood, C., Munn, Z. and Porritt, K. 2015. Qualitative research synthesis: Methodological guidance for systematic reviewers utilizing meta-aggregation. *International Journal of Evidence-Based Healthcare*, 13, 179–187.

Lord, B. and Woollard, M. 2011. The reliability of vital signs in estimating pain severity among adult patients treated by paramedics. *Emergency Medicine Journal*, 28, 147–150.

Lord, B., Bendall, J. and Reinten, T. 2014. The influence of paramedic and patient gender on the administration of analgesics in the out-of-hospital setting. *Prehospital Emergency Care*, 18, 195–200.

Mehra, M. R. et al. 2020. Retracted: Hydroxychloroquine or chloroquine with or without a macrolide for treatment of Covid-19: A multinational registry analysis. *The Lancet* (withdrawn article in press).

Middleton, P. M. et al. 2010. Effectiveness of morphine, fentanyl, and methoxyflurane in the prehospital setting. *Prehospital Emergency Care*, 14, 439–447.

National Institute for Health and Care Excellence (NICE). 2020. Healthcare databases advanced search. London: NICE. Available at: https://hdas.nice.org.uk/ [Accessed 12 December 2020].

Nguyen, A. and Catalan, D. 2020. Digital mis/disinformation and public engagment with health and science controversies: Fresh perspectives from Covid-19. *Media and Communication*, 8, 323–328.

Olasveengen, T. M., Prescott, R. J. and Kramer-Johansen, J. 2015. Impedance Threshold Device (ITD) during cardiac arrest – Does it work or not? *Resuscitation*, 94, A3–A4.

Olaussen, A. et al. 2017. Paramedic literature search filters: Optimised for clinicians and academics. *BMC Medical Informatics and Decision Making*, 17, 146.

Osuna, A. and Perez, A. 2020. Resolution of abnormal pulse oximetry measured in real-time in a neonate with vertebral subluxation: A case report. *Journal of Pediatric, Maternal and Family Health, Chiropractic*, 41–45.

Richardson, W. S. et al. 1995. The well-built clinical question: A key to evidence-based decisions. *ACP Journal Club*, 123, A12–13.

Soar, J. et al. 2015. European Resuscitation Council guidelines for resuscitation 2015: Section 3. Adult advanced life support. *Resuscitation*, 95, 100–147.

Trump, D. 2020. Hydroxychloroquine and azithromycin [Twitter]. Available at: https://twitter.com/ [Accessed 23 March 2020, account now closed].

Vincent, R. 1997. Drugs in modern resuscitation. *British Journal of Anaesthesia*, 79, 188–197.

Von Elm, E. et al. 2007. Strengthening the reporting of observational studies in epidemiology (STROBE) statement: Guidelines for reporting observational studies. *BMJ*, 335, 806–808.

Wang, C.-H. et al. 2015. Active compression-decompression resuscitation and impedance threshold device for out-of-hospital cardiac arrest: A systematic review and metaanalysis of randomized controlled trials. *Critical Care Medicine*, 43, 889–896.

Yannopoulos, D. et al. 2015. Quality of CPR: An important effect modifier in cardiac arrest clinical outcomes and intervention effectiveness trials. *Resuscitation*, 94, 106–113.

Chapter 10

Quality Improvement

David M. Williams

> ### *Chapter Objectives*
>
> This chapter will cover:
>
> - The roots of quality improvement in the ambulance service
> - The theoretical and practical foundations of the science of improvement
> - An operational definition of quality improvement
> - What makes a project a quality improvement project
> - Distinguishing enumerative from analytic studies
> - The key components of improvement projects, including chartering, tools, methods and measurement
> - Contextual factors that support successful improvement

Introduction

Quality improvement (QI) occurs through informal actions as part of day-to-day operations and structured approaches as planned improvement efforts. The learning generated about problems in practice, discoveries in developing and testing changes and the results achieved are a valuable contribution to the profession. QI shares attributes of design, measurement and change with traditional research but is also unique in its aim and execution. QI practised with rigour and fidelity can add knowledge to better enhance the profession's understanding of what works and to aid in adopting and implementing **evidence-based practices**.

Roots of Quality

The emergence of quality and the methods in use today are often attributed to American leaders working with the Japanese after the Second World War. Interest in designing and developing quality traces back far earlier (Juran, 1995). As industry focused more on mass production, increasing output and reducing costs to increase profit, leaders increasingly focused on designing processes to get better results more predictably.

Students of management are introduced to Frederick Taylor's *Scientific Management* at the turn of the 20th century (Taylor, 1911). Innovation followed in the 1920s with Henry Ford's publication of the concept of mass production through a new approach known as the assembly line. Many countries were learning about these techniques and trialling them in their companies.

After the Second World War, several Americans, including W. Edwards Deming, Joseph Juran and others, were invited to Japan and shared ideas of statistical thinking, scientific problem-solving and management principles grounded in quality. Japanese leaders adopted and built on many of these ideas, and quality in Japanese products improved to the world's attention. It wasn't until the 1980s that American industry took notice and began to adopt the principles and practices of leaders like Drs Deming and Juran and others from Japan.

Leaders in healthcare were among the curious and wondered how these principles could help, and they began to learn and apply them in the healthcare environment. Demonstration projects, early application and sharing of learning have shifted into a continually evolving focus of quality in healthcare and its many sectors (Berwick et al., 1990).

Science of Improvement (Perla et al., 2013)

Improvement science or the science of improvement emerged in healthcare and education as a descriptive term in improvement. Langley et al. (2009) introduced the phrasing 'the science of improvement'.

Knowledge is in two forms. First is the subject matter knowledge we each have from our trade and university studies and lived experience as practitioners of our profession. This knowledge is essential but not sufficient to improve, and the second body of knowledge is helpful for change. This body of knowledge framed by Dr Edwards Deming as the 'system of profound knowledge' includes: appreciating systems, understanding variation, theory of knowledge and psychology of change (Deming, 1993). Langley et al. (2009) defined the science of improvement as the interaction of these four lenses to improve performance. The application requires integrating a set of tools and methods with subject matter expertise to develop, test, implement and spread changes (Associates in Process Improvement, 2021a).

Many uses of the term 'improvement science' do not include the foundation in Deming's system of profound knowledge. Often the focus is only on the tools and methods of improvement at the project level or when applying the tool or method (that is, Plan-Do-Study-Act (PDSA) cycle, run charts).

Defining Quality Improvement

For our purposes, quality is the definition of what good looks like to the customer or patient. It is the desired result that any process or product produces to meet the need of a customer or patient. Improvement of quality requires changing the process or product to obtain a different result that is better than the previous results.

There are three distinct features here:

1. There is an operational definition of what is quality for the customer or patient.

2. A change is made to the process or system that causes an improved result.

3. The improved result sustains over time, reflecting a new level of improved performance.

This definition is essential and will conflict with other definitions in use. The focus of attention of QI is on the process or the system and not on individuals. The intervention is a change to the process of interest and does not include activities like training, inspection or feedback. The result is measured over time to confirm a sustained new level of performance.

Quality Improvement and Research

Healthcare is an evidence-based practice. The care delivered is based on research showing confidence that an intervention or drug creates the desired effect. This confidence comes from established research methods like **randomised control trials (RCTs)**, where subjects are randomly assigned to an intervention group and a control group to reduce **bias** and compare to similar populations. RCTs are a current standard in medicine, but this is not the only approach to generating knowledge (Deaton and Cartwright, 2018). The choice of method should be guided by the questions being asked (Academy of Medical Sciences, 2017). Also, RCTs are not without bias (Krauss, 2018) and attempts to replicate them with real-world data have not reliably yielded similar results (Averitt et al., 2020; Bartlett et al., 2019).

In QI, studies are conducted for learning and understanding how to take action on the system of interest to change results into the future (Provost, 2011). Dr Edwards Deming (1975) classified two types of studies based on the target for action: enumerative and analytic studies.

An enumerative study involves taking action on the area that was studied. For example, an ambulance provider observes that paramedics co-located with a field supervisor who restocks narcotics have a higher rate of administration of narcotic pain medication. To explore this hypothesis, data on narcotic administration are analysed for the subgroup of paramedic ambulances that are co-located with a supervisor and those that are not. This is a 'hypothesis-generating study' and an example of an enumerative study. The system was considered static and was not changed, and the results of the difference were for the area of study and during the study period.

Analytic studies are acting on the causal system to improve the results of the system of interest. For example, an ambulance trust tracked ambulance offloads at an emergency department over the previous 26 weeks using a Shewhart chart. The offload times were not acceptable to the system, but the data showed they were consistent over time. A test of change was developed to place a staff person onsite during peak hours to decontaminate, restock and otherwise help crews return to service. In the weeks following the intervention, average hospital offload times reduced to the desired level and sustained at that level. This study increased learning about the change, and the sustained results on the Shewhart chart increased the degree of belief that these results would sustain into the future. The learning also supported predicting similar results if the intervention were applied in other emergency departments with peak demands affecting handover times.

Studying Quality Improvement Methods Versus Applied Improvement

The study of QI may take different forms: studying the tools and methods or using the tools and methods to improve practice.

Studying the tools and methods themselves occurs when the focus of the study is on the tool or method. For example, QI researchers studied the use of the PDSA cycle by GP trainees as a strategy to support change management in their practices (Crowfoot and Prasad, 2017). The focus was on learning about the use of the method of PDSA and adds knowledge to the understanding of the QI methods.

Alternatively, improvers are focused on a theory of change to improve care delivery and use QI methods to accomplish the change. For example, improvers in Massachusetts, USA, wanted to improve the **outcomes** for patients with stroke-like presentations (Daudelin et al., 2013). The focus was on using an evidence-based care stroke bundle, and ambulance providers were part of a QI collaborative based on the IHI Breakthrough Series Model (Institute for Healthcare Improvement, 2003). QI methods were used to support them in testing the changes and measuring the results, but the area of focus was the care bundle.

In EMS research, improvement of practice or care delivery is the area of focus and QI tools and methods are the methodology used to enhance performance.

Institutional Review

In healthcare, the safety and privacy of patients are the priority in research and improvement. A common question is when and if an institutional (ethical) review is necessary or required for improvement work. The correct answer can vary by organisation. Many organisations establish criteria for improvement and institutional review board (IRB) review.

In 2003, the Hasting Center (Baily et al., 2006) began convening leaders from healthcare and improvement to understand the ethical considerations of QI and the protection of human subjects. With a shared purpose of protecting patients, QI was recognised as unique from research due to its routine presence in daily operations, its alignment with patients' desires for positive outcomes and its focus on supporting the implementation of new evidence using tools and methods of change (Lynn et al., 2007).

The group did note that patient harm is possible in QI, and so improvers must be conscious in their design and institutions may, in certain circumstances, consider an ethical review. Included were seven ethical requirements for protecting human participants in QI activities (see **Table 10.1**) (Emanuel et al., 2000).

If a policy is not in place, improvers should collaborate with their local IRB to establish standard criteria. IRBs benefit from having members who are experienced

Table 10.1 – Ethical requirements for the protection of human participants in quality improvement activities.

Requirements	Explanation
Social or scientific value	The gains from QI activity should justify the resources spent and the risks imposed on participants.
Scientific validity	A QI activity should be methodologically sound (i.e. properly structured to achieve the goals).
Fair participant selection	Participants should be selected to achieve a fair distribution of the burdens and benefits of QI.
Favourable risk–benefit ratio	A QI activity should be designed to limit risks while maximising potential benefits and to ensure the risks to an individual human participant are balanced by expected benefits to the participants and to society.
Respect for the participants	A QI activity should be designed to protect the privacy of participants and the confidentiality of personal information. Participants in a QI activity should receive information about findings from the activity that are clinically relevant to their own care. All patients and workers in a care delivery setting should receive basic information about the programme of QI activities. The QI results should be freely shared with others in the healthcare system, but participant confidentiality should be protected by putting results into a non-identifiable form or obtaining specific consent to share.

(continued)

Table 10.1 – Ethical requirements for the protection of human participants in quality improvement activities. (*continued*)

Requirements	Explanation
Informed consent	Consent to inclusion in minimal-risk QI activities is part of the patient's consent to receive treatment.
	Patients should be asked for **informed consent** to be included in a specific QI activity if the activity imposes more than minimal risk.
	The risk to patients should be measured relative to the risk associated with receiving standard healthcare.
	Workers (employees or nonemployee professionals who provide care in the organisation) should participate in minimal-risk QI activities as part of their job responsibilities.
	Workers should be asked for informed consent to be included in a QI activity that imposes more than minimal risk.
	The risk to workers should be measured relative to the risk associated with the usual work situation. This does not include any risk to economic security (for example, if a QI activity reveals that the worker is incompetent or that the organisation can provide care without the worker).
Independent review	Accountability for the clinical conduct of QI should be integrated into the practices that ensure accountability for clinical care.
	Each QI activity should receive the kind of ethical review and supervision that is appropriate to its level of potential risk and project worth.

Source: Emanuel et al. (2000).

and knowledgeable in improvement and research. Full IRB review of QI work is not routine, and submissions are commonly returned exempt. If there is any question of whether IRB review is required or if there is intent to submit the work for publication to a peer-reviewed journal, submission to IRB is recommended.

Quality Improvement Projects

QI projects are distinct from other types of projects or activities. QI projects have a defined outcome for improvement, and the work includes testing changes to a process or system to enhance the results. Many projects described in trade publications, conference sessions and even peer-reviewed publications as QI projects or initiatives do not meet these definitions of QI.

The following are examples of improvement projects for paramedic care and ambulance systems:

- Improve the identification of deteriorating patients.

- Reduce time from onset of symptoms in a patient with a suspected ST-segment elevation myocardial infraction (STEMI) to performing percutaneous coronary intervention (PCI) to 90 minutes or less.

- Improve identification and rapid notification of suspected sepsis patients.

- Reduce hospital turnaround time at the emergency department.

- Reduce the number of patients transported who are discharged from the emergency department on the same day.

The following are typical examples that are not good examples of QI projects:

- Campaign to increase the awareness of paramedics of the elements of the stroke bundle.

- Retrospectively audit patients intubated by paramedics to confirm protocol compliance.

- Give feedback to individual paramedics on individual cases with or without error or harm.

- Collect and report individual paramedic statistics compared to peer caregivers.

- Hold training programmes to refresh paramedics on care conditions or protocols that are not currently meeting compliance goals.

- Perform peer reviews of individual cases with suspected caregiver error or patient harm.

These activities are not considered QI because there is no clear definition of improvement, and the area of focus is not to change the process to produce a different result. Sample audits, training and feedback can be factors within a change theory but are not process changes alone. Individual feedback, benchmarking of caregivers and peer review can result in tampering and produce a culture that is not supportive of improvement and patient safety.

Chartering Improvement Initiatives

Improvement work is framed using a 'consistent, structured approach that affords a common language' (Langley et al., 2009), also known as a framework or roadmap. In healthcare, the Model for Improvement is widely used. The Model for Improvement includes three questions that act as the foundation for the chartering of an improvement project:

1. What are we trying to accomplish (aim statement and outcome)?

2. How will we know a change is an improvement (feedback or measurement system)?

3. What changes can we make that will result in improvement (change theory)?

Also included is the PDSA cycle, emphasising the value of testing to learn. The answers to these three questions provide the basis of an improvement charter. **Box 10.1** shows a checklist to assess and improve a project charter (Associates in Process Improvement, 2021b).

Box 10.1 A Checklist to Support Assessment and an Improvement Project Charter

WHAT ARE WE TRYING TO ACCOMPLISH? Aim and rationale

- The charter relates to the organisation's strategic plans/objectives.
- The charter description clearly states the need for improvement.
- The expected impact to the organisation is clear (clinical outcomes, cycle time, financial and so forth).
- The improvement clearly points to process, product, service or sub-system improvement.
- The impact on the patient or external customer is clear.
- The expected outcomes are clear and the team will know when it has completed the project.
- There are specific, numerical goals to be attained.
- The project can be completed within a timeframe.

HOW WILL WE KNOW A CHANGE IS AN IMPROVEMENT?

- An appropriate family of measures is identified.
- Measures identified are directly related to the project description, objectives and goals.
- Historical data exist on the performance of the process or product to be improved.
- Outcome, process and balancing measures are specified.
- Measures can be collected at intervals frequent enough to assess progress on the project.

- Improvement in the project measures can reasonably be expected within the project timeframe.
- The financial impact is easily calculated and supported by the organisation's financial group.

WHAT CHANGES CAN WE MAKE THAT WILL RESULT IN IMPROVEMENT? Initial cycles, boundaries, other guidance

- Specific issues to investigate and/or alternatives to consider are given.
- A concept design or change package is identified.
- Project constraints are defined, including what is NOT to be addressed.
- The objectives clearly state that the team can develop, test and implement changes.
- Project is tied to specific processes or sub-systems.
- Initial activities or PDSA cycles are suggested.

PARTICIPATION: Team membership

- All appropriate subject matter knowledge is represented on the improvement team.
- Process owner (with authority to make changes) is represented or a sponsor of the team.
- People with detailed knowledge of the targeted system are on the team.
- Patients, customers or suppliers are on the team.

Each bullet may be assessed on a Likert scale, with 1 being not present and 5 being fully present. Any item less than 5 is an opportunity to improve the design of the improvement project.

Contextual Factors Affecting the Success of a QI Project

In addition to the technical factors included in a QI charter, there are contextual factors that can contribute to the success of a QI project (Kaplan et al., 2012). A Model for Understanding Success In Quality (MUSIQ) was developed that considers 25 contextual factors to consider to improve the success of a QI effort.

The contextual factors identified fall into six broad categories:

1. External environment
2. Organisation
3. QI support and capacity

4. Microsystem

5. QI team

6. Miscellaneous.

This model has been tested with various improvement initiatives, and additional recommendations for contextual factors have been recommended (Reed et al., 2018). The MUSIQ assessment aids understanding of the contextual factors to support successful improvement work. It provides guidance in concert with the charter checklist and SQUIRE 2.0 guidelines to improve the design of QI projects.

Measurement for Improvement

The example just described includes the use of time series data and analytic tools like run (Perla et al., 2011) or Shewhart charts. Collecting outcome and process measurements in time series and displaying in a run or Shewhart chart is best practice in QI. **Figure 10.1** is an example of a Shewhart chart.

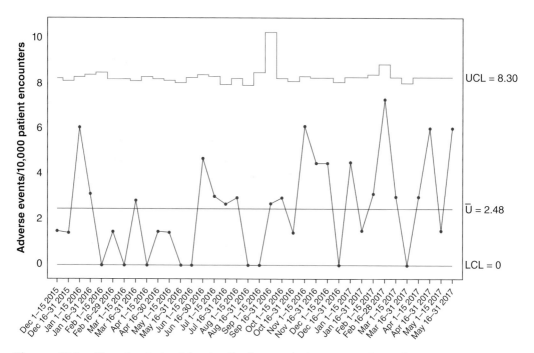

Figure 10.1 – Shewhart chart (u-chart) of an ambulance service adverse event rate.
Source: Howard et al. (2018).

Measurement for improvement is different from measurement used for accountability and research and is used as a continuous vital sign in parallel to making changes to the process or system (Solberg et al., 1997). Data are displayed visually in time order to determine if a change is an improvement and to distinguish between common cause variation (stable variation) and special cause variation (attributable causes) (Berwick, 1991).

Common QI Tools and Methods

QI includes many tools and methods. A tool is a 'technique, object or device for completing a specific task', and a method is a 'broader procedure or approach to accomplishing something following a specific plan of a set of tools' (Langley et al., 2009). The tools and methods for improvement can be organised into the following six categories:

1. Viewing systems and processes

2. Gathering information

3. Organising information

4. Understanding variation

5. Understanding relationships

6. Managing projects.

Table 10.2 is a summary of common tools and methods in each category.

Documenting QI for Publication

In 2005, healthcare improvers believed in the importance of publishing QI work in peer-reviewed journals, and limited guidance existed to support the framing of QI work. The result was the publication of what is now known as the SQUIRE guidelines or the Standards for QUality Improvement Reporting Excellence (Davidoff and Batalden, 2005). The guidelines were updated to version 2.0 in 2015 (Ogrinc et al., 2016).

The SQUIRE 2.0 guidelines aid authors to consider additional QI context when reporting using the standard sections of a traditional journal paper. **Table 10.3** is a summary of the reporting method.

The SQUIRE 2.0 guidance can be helpful when starting a QI initiative to support proper chartering and data collection. It can also serve as a checklist to support the execution and documentation of the learning and results of a QI project. It is recommended to consider the guidelines at the start of any QI work and incorporate them into the project's design.

Table 10.2 – Tools and methods of improvement.

Category	Methods	Tools
Viewing systems and processes	Process mapping Dynamic simulation	Flow diagrams Causal loop diagrams Linkage of processes
Gathering information	Surveys Benchmarking Creativity methods	Data collection form Operational definitions
Organising information	Quality function deployment Failure mode effectiveness analysis Problem solving	Affinity diagrams Force-field analysis Cause-and-affect diagram Driver diagram Matrix diagram Tree diagram Interrelationship diagram Radar chart
Understanding variation	Statistical process control Measurement system analysis Statistical methods	Run chart Frequency plot Pareto chart Shewhart control chart Other graphs
Understanding relationships	Planned experimentation	Scatter plot Two-way table
Managing projects	Model for improvement PDSA cycle	Gantt chart PERT chart Work breakdown structure A3 diagram

Source: Adapted from Langley et al. (2009).

Table 10.3 – Revised standards for quality improvement reporting excellence (SQUIRE 2.0) publication guidelines.

Text Section and Item Name	Section or Item Description
Title and abstract	
1. Title	Indicate that the manuscript concerns an initiative to improve healthcare (broadly defined to include the quality, safety, effectiveness, patient-centredness, timeliness, cost, efficiency and equity of healthcare).
2. Abstract	a Provide adequate information to aid in searching and indexing. b Summarise all key information from various sections of the text using the abstract format of the intended publication or a structured summary such as: background, local problem, methods, interventions, results, conclusions.
Introduction	*Why did you start?*
3. Problem description	Nature and significance of the local problem.
4. Available knowledge	Summary of what is currently known about the problem, including relevant previous studies.
5. Rationale	Informal or formal frameworks, models, concepts and/or theories used to explain the problem, any reasons or assumptions that were used to develop the intervention(s) and reasons why the intervention(s) was expected to work.
Methods	*What did you do?*
6. Specific aims	Purpose of the project and of this report.
7. Context	Contextual elements considered important at the outset of introducing the intervention(s).
8. Intervention(s)	a Description of the intervention(s) in sufficient detail that others could reproduce it. b Specifics of the team involved in the work.
9. Study of the intervention(s)	a Approach chosen for assessing the impact of the intervention(s). b Approach used to establish whether the observed outcomes were due to the intervention(s).

(*continued*)

Table 10.3 – Revised standards for quality improvement reporting excellence (SQUIRE 2.0) publication guidelines. (*continued*)

Text Section and Item Name	Section or Item Description
10. Measures	a Measures chosen for studying processes and outcomes of the intervention(s), including rationale for choosing them, their operational definitions and their **validity** and **reliability**. b Description of the approach to the ongoing assessment of contextual elements that contributed to the success, failure, efficiency and cost. c Methods employed for assessing completeness and accuracy of data.
11. Analysis	Qualitative and quantitative methods used to draw inferences from the data. Methods for understanding variation within the data, including the effects of time as a variable.
12. Ethical considerations	Ethical aspects of implementing and studying the intervention(s) and how they were addressed, including, but not limited to, formal ethics review and potential conflict(s) of interest.
Results	*What did you find?*
13. Results	a Initial steps of the intervention(s) and their evolution over time (for example, time-line diagram, flow chart or table), including modifications made to the intervention during the project. b Details of the process measures and outcomes. c Contextual elements that interacted with the intervention(s). d Observed associations between outcomes, interventions and relevant contextual elements. e Unintended consequences such as unexpected benefits, problems, failures or costs associated with the intervention(s). f Details about missing data.
Discussion	*What does it mean?*
14. Summary	a Key findings, including relevance to the rationale and specific aims. b Particular strengths of the project.

Text Section and Item Name	Section or Item Description
15. Interpretation	a Nature of the association between the intervention(s) and the outcomes. b Comparison of results with findings from other publications. c Impact of the project on people and systems. d Reasons for any differences between observed and anticipated outcomes, including the influence of context. e Costs and strategic trade-offs, including opportunity costs.
16. Limitations	a Limits to the **generalisability** of the work. b Factors that might have limited internal validity such as confounding bias or imprecision in the design. c Methods, measurement or analysis. d Efforts made to minimise and adjust for limitations.
17. Conclusions	a Usefulness of the work. b Sustainability. c Potential for spread to other contexts. d Implications for practice and for further study in the field. e Suggested next steps.
Other information	
18. Funding	Sources of funding that supported this work. Role, if any, of the funding organisation in the design, implementation, interpretation and reporting.

Source: Adapted from Ogrinc et al. (2016).

Practical Examples of QI in Peer-reviewed Publications

There is a lack of peer-reviewed published EMS QI projects with the rigour and fidelity seen in the quality and healthcare literature. Here are three examples of note.

The Massachusetts Emergency Medical Service Stroke Quality Improvement Collaborative, 2009–2012 (Daudelin et al., 2013)

Using a shared approach and focused on stroke, 17 EMS agencies across Massachusetts, USA, participated in a Breakthrough Series Collaborative. Sponsored by the Massachusetts Department of Health, participants used tools and methods like PDSA testing and run chart measurement across a family of measures and participated in quarterly learning sessions and coaching calls. All five process measures tracked over the collaborative noted improvement and reached 90% or better.

Ambulance Trigger Tool for Adverse Events

Hamad Ambulance Service at Hamad Medical Corporation is the national ambulance service provider for the country of Qatar. Consultant paramedics, inspired by the IHI Global Trigger Tool (GTT) (Griffin and Resar, 2009) used in hospital to measure adverse events and harm, worked with the Institute for Healthcare Improvement to develop prototype triggers designed around potential harm in the ambulance setting (Howard et al., 2017). These triggers were applied to more than 80,000 encounters. Mirroring the sample, review, data collection and measuring process of the GTT, consultant paramedics tested the ambulance trigger tool for 20 consecutive samples (Howard et al., 2018). The results of their review with the tool were reported in Shewhart charts.

Enhancing CPR During Transition From Prehospital to Emergency Department: A QI Initiative (Hoehn et al., 2020)

High-quality CPR with limited interruption is a critical factor in the survival of paediatric out-of-hospital cardiac arrest. Emergency physicians in a paediatric emergency department aimed to decrease pauses in compression from 17 seconds to 10 seconds in the first 2 minutes of care. Secondary aims were to have no pause longer than 10 seconds and have all encounters with time to pad placement in less than 120 seconds. The team developed a key driver diagram of their theory of change and tested their theory iteratively across 33 encounters. The QI project resulted in decreased interruptions to 12 seconds in the first 2 minutes and 7 seconds for any pause after. There was a reduction of variation in pad application. Their reporting included their key driver diagram and annotated Shewhart charts for crucial process measures.

Summary

Quality improvement projects are vital activities for developing knowledge about ambulance services and paramedic care, learning what works and what doesn't and enhancing performance. The tools and methods of the science of improvement joined with subject matter knowledge and expertise result in breakthrough improvement. The ambulance service has a long history of deep interest in quality but is still a novice in adopting and executing rigorous QI with fidelity. QI tools and methods offer an opportunity for leaders to learn and improve. Well-designed and executed improvement projects should be reported in peer-reviewed journals and shared across this profession. This chapter introduces the methodology and potential.

Further Reading

Langley, G. J. et al. 2009. *The Improvement Guide: A Practical Approach to Enhancing Organizational Performance*, 2nd Edn. San Francisco, Jossey-Bass.

Provost, L.P. and Murray, S.K. 2011. *The Health Care Data Guide: Learning from Data for Improvement*, 63. San Francisco, Jossey-Bass.

Swor, R. 2005. *Quality Management in Prehospital Care*, 2nd Edn. National Association of EMS Physicians.

US Department of Transportation, National Highway Traffic Safety Administration. 1997. *Leadership Guide to Quality Improvement for Emergency Medical Services (EMS) Systems*. US Government, Washington DC.

References

Academy of Medical Sciences. 2017. Sources of evidence for assessing the safety, efficacy, and effectiveness of medicines. Available at: https://acmedsci.ac.uk/file-download/86466482 [Accessed 5 January 2021].

Associates in Process Improvement. 2021a. API definition of the science of improvement. Available at: http://www.apiweb.org/media/mod_jmslideshow/900x439_fill_slide02_new.jpg [Accessed 5 January 2021].

Associates in Process Improvement. 2021b. Improvement project charter assessment feedback form. Available at: http://www.ihi.org/resources/Pages/Tools/QI-Project-Charter.aspx [Accessed 5 January 2021].

Averitt, A. J. et al. 2020. Translating evidence into practice: Eligibility criteria fail to eliminate clinically significant differences between real-world and study populations. *NPJ Digital Medicine*, 3, 67.

Baily, M. A. et al. 2006. The ethics of using QI methods to improve health care quality and safety. *Hastings Center Report*, 36, S1–S40.

Bartlett, V. L. et al. 2019. Feasibility of using real-world data to replicate clinical trial evidence. *JAMA Network Open*, 2, e1912869.

Berwick, D. M. 1991. Controlling variation in health care: A consultation from Walter Shewhart. *Medical Care*, 29, 1212–1225.

Berwick, D. M., Godfrey, A. B. and Roessner, J. 1990. *Curing Health Care: New Strategies for Quality Improvement*. San Francisco, Wiley.

Crowfoot, D. and Prasad, V. 2017. Using the plan-do-study-act (PDSA) cycle to make change in general practice. *InnovAiT*, 10, 425–430.

Daudelin, D. H. et al. 2013. The Massachusetts Emergency Medical Service Stroke Quality Improvement Collaborative, 2009–2012. *Preventing Chronic Disease*, 10, E161.

Davidoff, F. and Batalden, P. 2005. Toward stronger evidence on quality improvement. Draft publication guidelines: The beginning of a consensus project. *Quality and Safety in Health Care*, 14, 319–325.

Deaton, A. and Cartwright, N. 2018. Understanding and misunderstanding randomized controlled trials. *Social Science and Medicine*, 210, 2–21.

Deming, W. E. 1975. On probability as a basis for action. *The American Statistician*, 29, 146–152.

Deming, W. E. 1993. *The New Economics*. Cambridge, Massachusetts Institute of Technology.

Emanuel, E. J., Wendler, D. and Grady, C. 2000. What makes clinical research ethical? *JAMA*, 283, 2701–2711.

Griffin, F. A. and Resar, R. K. 2009. *IHI global trigger tool for measuring adverse events* (2nd Edn). IHI Innovation Series white paper. Cambridge, Institute for Healthcare Improvement.

Hoehn, E. F. et al. 2020. Enhancing CPR during transition from prehospital to emergency department: A QI initiative. *Pediatrics*, 145, e20192908.

Howard, I. et al. 2018. Application of the emergency medical services trigger tool to measure adverse events in prehospital emergency care: A time series analysis. *BMC Emergency Medicine*, 18, 47.

Howard, I. L. et al. 2017. Development of a trigger tool to identify adverse events and harm in Emergency Medical Services. *Emergency Medicine Journal*, 34, 391–397.

Institute for Healthcare Improvement. 2003. *The Breakthrough Series: IHI's Collaborative Model for Achieving Breakthrough Improvement*. Cambridge, IHI.

Juran, J. 1995. *A History of Managing for Quality*. Milwaukee, ASQC/Quality Press.

Kaplan, H. C. et al. 2012. The Model for Understanding Success in Quality (MUSIQ): Building a theory of context in healthcare quality improvement. *BMJ Quality and Safety*, 21, 13–20.

Krauss, A. 2018. Why all randomised controlled trials produce biased results. *Annals of Medicine*, 50, 312–322.

Langley, G. J. et al. 2009. *The Improvement Guide: A Practical Approach to Enhancing Organizational Performance*, 2nd Edn. San Francisco, Jossey-Bass.

Lynn, J. et al. 2007. The ethics of using quality improvement methods in health care. *Annals of Internal Medicine*, 146, 666–673.

Ogrinc, G. et al. 2016. SQUIRE 2.0 (Standards for QUality Improvement Reporting Excellence): Revised publication guidelines from a detailed consensus process. *BMJ Quality and Safety*, 25, 986–992.

Perla, R. J., Provost, L. P. and Murray, S. K. 2011. The run chart: A simple analytical tool for learning from variation in healthcare processes. *BMJ Quality and Safety*, 20, 46–51.

Perla, R. J., Provost, L. P. and Parry, G. J. 2013. Seven propositions of the science of improvement: Exploring foundations. *Quality Management in Health Care*, 22, 170–186.

Provost, L. P. 2011. Analytical studies: A framework for quality improvement design and analysis. *BMJ Quality and Safety*, 20, i92–i96.

Reed, J. E., Kaplan, H. C. and Ismail, S. A. 2018. A new typology for understanding context: Qualitative exploration of the model for understanding success in quality (MUSIQ). *BMC Health Services Research*, 18, 584.

Solberg, L. I., Mosser, G. and McDonald, S. 1997. The three faces of performance measurement: Improvement, accountability, and research. *Joint Commission Journal on Quality Improvement*, 23, 135–147.

Taylor, F. W. 1911. *The Principles of Scientific Management*. New York, Harper and Brothers Publishers.

Glossary

Action research: Research involving healthcare practitioners conducting systematic enquiries in order to help them improve their own practices, which in turn can enhance their working environment and the working environments of clients, patients and service users.

Axiology: The branch of philosophy concerned with the study of principles and values, related to ethics and aesthetics.

Before-and-after study: A quasi-experimental study in which the dependent variable (outcome of interest) is measured before the intervention is implemented (control phase) and after it has been implemented (intervention phase).

Bias: Any systematic error in a study that results in an incorrect estimate of the true effect of an exposure on the outcome of interest.

Boolean operators: Words such as AND, OR, NOT, that connect search terms to create a logical phrase that a database is designed to understand.

Case-control study: An observational study in which participants with and without a condition of interest (outcome) are identified and data on risk factors or exposures are analysed to see which of these affect the outcome.

Case study research: A qualitative, mixed or multi-method approach in which the researcher explores a bounded system or systems over time, collecting in-depth data from multiple sources such as observations, interviews, audio-visual material, documents and reports.

Chart review: Studies in which information is abstracted from the medical records, whether paper or electronic, and analysed to explore relationships between risk factors (exposures) and outcomes.

Clinical audit: The measurement of quality of care over time against well-defined standards.

Cohort study: An observational study in which participants exposed to different risk factors are followed over time, to determine whether one or more exposure affects an outcome of interest.

Concurrent designs: Methods are undertaken at the same time.

Confidence interval: Probability that a population parameter will fall between a set of values for a certain proportion of times.

Confounding: Distortion of the association between an exposure and outcome of interest by an extraneous third variable (called a confounder).

Confounder: An alternative explanation for an association between an exposure and outcome of interest.

Consensus methods: Formal systematic research designs for groups (stakeholders) to reach agreement, where possible, on areas of uncertainty.

Consensus development conference: The consensus development conference or panel is a group of selected experts with a chairperson for producing consensus statements on the benefits, costs, adverse effects and research gaps related to medical interventions or health technologies including drugs, devices and procedures.

Consolidated Standards of Reporting Trials (CONSORT): Guidelines developed as a framework to improve the reporting of randomised controlled trials.

Constructivism/interpretivism: Considers that there are multiple realities relative to each individual, and that knowledge is subjective (subjectivism) and co-constructed between participant and researcher.

Critical appraisal: The process of carefully and systematically examining research to judge its trustworthiness, and its value and relevance in a particular context.

Critical Appraisal Skills Programme (CASP): Tools for assessing risk of bias of research studies.

Cross-sectional study: An observational study that analyses population data at one specific point or during a specific period in time, to allow estimation of prevalence of a given condition, service or other outcome and relationships with other factors or exposures.

Delphi method: A type of consensus method where repeated surveys are distributed to a group of key informants designed to generate and prioritise ideas.

Enrol: To include a person or participant in a research study.

Epistemology: The branch of philosophy concerned with the nature of knowledge.

The Enhancing the QUAlity and Transparency Of health Research network (EQUATOR): An international initiative seeking to improve the reliability and value of published health research by promoting transparent and accurate reporting.

Equipoise: Uncertainty as to which treatment pathway leads to improved patient outcomes.

Ethnography: A type of qualitative research design, often involving observations or interviews, which aims to understand people's cultures, beliefs and values through immersion of the researcher in a given community or environment, ideally over an extended period of time.

Evidence-based practice: The conscientious, explicit and judicious use of current best evidence, combined with clinician experience and patient preferences and values, when making decisions about the care of individual patients.

External validity/generalisability: The ability to generalise study findings to other contexts (populations, settings).

Feasibility study: A study undertaken to determine if a piece of research is feasible, not to answer a specific clinical question.

Generalisability/external validity: The ability to generalise study findings to other contexts (populations, settings).

Good Clinical Practice (GCP): The international ethical, scientific and practical standard to which all clinical research is conducted.

Grading of Recommendations Assessment, Development and Evaluation (GRADE): Systems for assessing how much confidence to place in findings from quantitative evidence syntheses.

Grading of Recommendations Assessment, Development and Evaluation and Confidence in the Evidence from Reviews of QUALitative research (GRADE-CERQual): Systems for assessing how much confidence to place in findings from qualitative evidence syntheses.

Grounded theory: A type of qualitative research design that is inductive in nature and involves collecting and analysing data in order to build theory.

Hierarchy of evidence: A ranking of study designs based on the rigour (strength and precision) of their research methods in making causal inferences.

Informed consent: When a person with mental capacity, after having received all necessary information, volunteers to participate in research.

Integration: The process of describing the relationships, links or interactions between the quantitative and qualitative components of a mixed methods study.

Internal consistency: The extent to which items in a questionnaire or scale are correlated with each other.

Internal validity: The extent to which what a study purports to show is true.

Interpretivism/constructivism: Considers that there are multiple realities relative to each individual, and that knowledge is subjective (subjectivism) and co-constructed between participant and researcher.

Inter-rater reliability: The degree of concordance between separate observations of the same phenomenon taken by different observers or raters.

Interrupted time series: A quasi-experimental design where several measurements are taken before and after the implementation of an intervention in order to determine the intervention effect over a period of time.

Mental capacity: The ability to make decisions for oneself, assessed as the ability understand, retain, weigh and use information to make decisions.

Meta-analysis: A statistical technique for combining numerical data from multiple quantitative studies.

Meta-inference: A conclusion (or conclusions) that encompass the different components of a mixed methods study.

Meta-integration: A technique used to combine the findings from a quantitative and a qualitative synthesis.

Meta-synthesis: An integrative technique to combine non-numerical data from multiple qualitative studies.

Mixed methods research: At least one quantitative method and one qualitative in the same study.

Multiple methods: A study with more than one quantitative method (for example, survey and analysis of records) or more than one qualitative method (for example, focus groups and interviews).

Narrative synthesis: Non-numerical analysis of the overall findings within a systematic review.

Nominal group technique: A type of consensus method approach, involving a structured, facilitated face-to-face meeting of key informants designed to generate ideas independently, agree a composite list of the most relevant ideas through discussion and refinement in a group or subgroups of participants and then to rate, rank or vote to prioritise the ideas put forward, in two (or sometimes more) rounds to achieve a consensus.

Nuremberg Code: A set of ethical principles for human research created as a result of the Nuremberg trials following the Second World War.

Observational study: Research including cohort, cross-sectional and case-control studies, which involves collection and analysis of patient data without the investigator altering treatments or pathways of care.

Ontology: The branch of philosophy concerned with the nature of reality.

Outcome: Measure of effectiveness, such as patient mortality, recurrence of event, hospital stay or patient experience.

Paramedic PhD: International registry of doctorates in the field of paramedicine (https://www.paramedicphd.com/).

Phase 1 study: Also termed a first-in-human study, seeks to assess safety and tolerability in healthy volunteers.

Phase 2 study: Sometimes termed an efficacy trial, aims to demonstrate proof of concept that a drug has a therapeutic effect and to identify the optimal dose, typically enrolling 100–500 patients.

Phase 3 study: Sometimes termed an effectiveness or confirmatory trial, sets out to confirm the safety and effectiveness of the drug in larger numbers (typically 1,000–5,000) of patients.

Phase 4 study: Focuses on the long-term safety surveillance and real-life performance of a drug in practice and can also explore additional indications where the drug may be effective.

Phenomenology: A type of qualitative research design that aims to understand the common meaning attached to a particular phenomenon by research participants who have experienced it.

Pilot study: A miniature version, either internal (data obtained form part of the analysis for the main trial) or external (data are analysed separately from the main trial), of the main trial which tests whether the components and processes of the main study (for example, to ensure recruitment, randomisation, treatment and follow-up assessments) all run smoothly together.

PICO: Population, Intervention, Comparator and Outcome; or for qualitative research.

PICo: Population, phenomena of Interest and Context.

Positivism: Conceives that there is one reality and it is apprehendable.

Postpositivism: Conceives that knowledge is subject to conjecture (an opinion or conclusion formed on the basis of incomplete information), and that replicated findings are probably true but are always subject to falsification.

Pragmatism: Commonly adopted in mixed methods research, emphasises the use of methods that work for the research questions, or where the utility of the research is highly valued.

Principlism: An approach to biomedical ethics which uses the four principles or 'Georgetown principles' of respect for autonomy (the ability to decide for oneself), non-maleficence (not doing harm), beneficence (doing good) and justice (acting fairly).

PRISMA: Preferred Reporting Items for Systematic reviews and Meta-Analyses.

Propensity score matching: A statistical technique that artificially creates control and intervention groups, from within a population of patients, some of whom received an intervention and some who did not.

Proposal: A brief summary of a proposed research study. It should provide an overview, including background, research question, aims and objectives, methods, ethical considerations and patient and public involvement and engagement.

PROSPERO: The International Prospective Register of Systematic Reviews.

Protocol: A full description of a research study which should act as a 'manual' for researchers to follow, including the evidence base and rationale, research question, hypothesis, study design and how the trial will be conducted, analysed and reported.

Quality improvement (QI): The informal actions as part of day-to-day operations and structured approaches as planned improvement efforts. It shares attributes of design, measurement and change with traditional research but is also unique in its aim and execution. Practised with rigour and fidelity, it can add knowledge to better enhance the profession's understanding of what works and aid in adopting and implementing evidence-based practices.

Quasi-experimental study: Non-randomised studies where outcomes are analysed by comparing groups by the treatments they received.

Randomisation: The process of randomly assigning a trial participant to the intervention or control group.

Randomised controlled trial (RCT): An experimental study in which one or more human subjects are prospectively assigned to one or more interventions (which may include placebo or other control) to evaluate the effects of those interventions on health-related biomedical or behavioural outcomes.

Rapid review: Evidence synthesis which accelerates the traditional systematic review process by streamlining or omitting methods to produce timely and efficient evidence.

Reliability: The consistency, or repeatability, of a measurement.

REporting of studies Conducted using Observational Routinely-collected Data (RECORD): Guidelines to promote transparent and accurate reporting of observational studies.

Research: The creative and systematic work undertaken in order to increase the stock of knowledge.

Research paradigm: A set of beliefs about research and how to undertake it.

Selection bias: When the wrong subjects or people are included, when subjects who should have been included are not or when the right data are collected but on the wrong people.

Sequential design: One method is undertaken after another is completed.

Service evaluation: A study to define or judge current care without reference to a standard within one healthcare service. A service evaluation is not typically considered formal research, but usually requires organisational approval.

SPICE: Setting, Perspective, Intervention, Comparison and Evaluation.

SPIDER: Sample, Phenomenon of Interest, Design, Evaluation, Research type.

Strengthening The Reporting of OBservational studies in Epidemiology (STROBE): Reporting guidelines to promote transparent and accurate reporting of observational studies.

Systematic review: A review of the evidence on a clearly formulated question that uses systematic and explicit methods to identify, select and critically appraise relevant primary research, and to extract and analyse data from the studies that are included in the review.

Triangulation: Looking at a phenomenon using different methods, and considering how findings agree, disagree and help to explain findings from other methods.

Validity: The extent to which a study shows what it purports to - internal validity refers to how the research findings match reality, while external validity refers to the extent to which the research findings are generalisable.

Waived consent: When a person without mental capacity is enrolled into a research study without consent.

Index

Note: Page numbers followed by *b* and *t* indicate box and tables respectively.

Index